A GUIDE TO GENTLE NUTRITION

Michelle Yandle

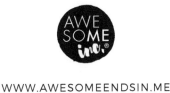

WWW.AWESOMEENDSIN.ME

A GUIDE TO GENTLE NUTRITION
BY MICHELLE YANDLE

Copyright © AwesoME Inc®
Written by Michelle Yandle for AwesoME Inc®
First published on www.AwesomeEndsIn.Me

ISBN 978-0-473-41967-7

Cover design & typeset by Nicole Perry
Cover image: Katie O'Neill

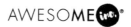

Published by ME Incorporated Limited T/A AwesoME Inc®
PO Box 95158, Swanson, Auckland 0653, New Zealand

WWW.AWESOMEENDSIN.ME

contents

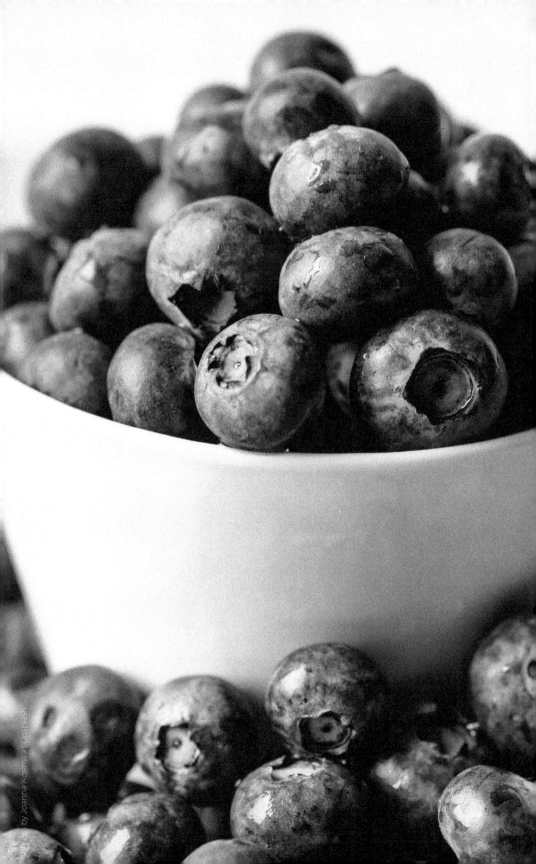

What is Gentle Nutrition?

An introduction.

There are so many rules out there when it comes to nutrition – everywhere you look, people are telling you to stop eating this or start eating that.

So many rules have been created that I am pretty sure there is not a food on the planet that hasn't been deemed dangerous at some point on the world-wide-web.

So what's a person to do?
I believe there should only be one 'rule' and that rule is, when it comes to nutrition, to start from a place of gratitude and self respect. Start by tuning out the dieting dogma and simply turn within. Thank your body for being there for you and ask it what it needs.

Have you ever asked your body what it actually wants?
Have you even asked if it is hungry before grabbing that biscuit or questioning what it really needs?

Our bodies are clever entities – they know what they need for energy, for endurance and overall performance. If you take the time to listen to your body's hunger rather than your head you'll find it has a lot of great suggestions.

Have you ever eaten fresh seasonal fruits or vegetables and felt bloated and lethargic? Have you ever had some fresh salmon or other fatty fish and wish you hadn't? Assuming of course, you didn't eat too much! Did that homemade muesli with coconut yogurt make you want to take a nap? Probably not.

Essentially, your body needs macro-nutrients such as fats and protein and micro-nutrients, those little vitamins and minerals that keep everything functioning.

Crowding those in as often as possible by simply revolving your meals around fresh produce, good quality natural proteins and healthy fats. Then you are giving your body exactly what it wants and needs, and THAT is the ultimate way of thanking your body for what it does for you.

Does your nutrition need to be strict? Does it need to be good 100% of the time?
No way! In fact eating in a way that allows for those occasional 'soul foods' has been shown over and over again to provide long term solutions to your health.

So where do you start?
When it comes to nutrition, think about the foods that make you feel the best physically AND mentally. Simply start by getting more of those! Sure there are some foods that make you happy short term but your body doesn't want a short term solution it wants to feel amazing always.

Before eating any meal, I encourage you to tune in and ask your body whether it is actually physically hungry and not just your head saying – eat that! Once you've done that, whether you're physically hungry or not, follow up with asking your body what it needs. It may be food, it may be comfort or entertainment. If it is food, load up on vegetables or fruit first, add some protein and then healthy fats. Do this as often as possible and then relax and enjoy the times in between where you might want something to sooth your soul rather than your physical body.

I want to share with you one of those recipes that sooth the body AND soul. These nutrient-dense muffins (recipe on next page) are moist and chocolatey and those hidden veggies will fool the pickiest of eaters.

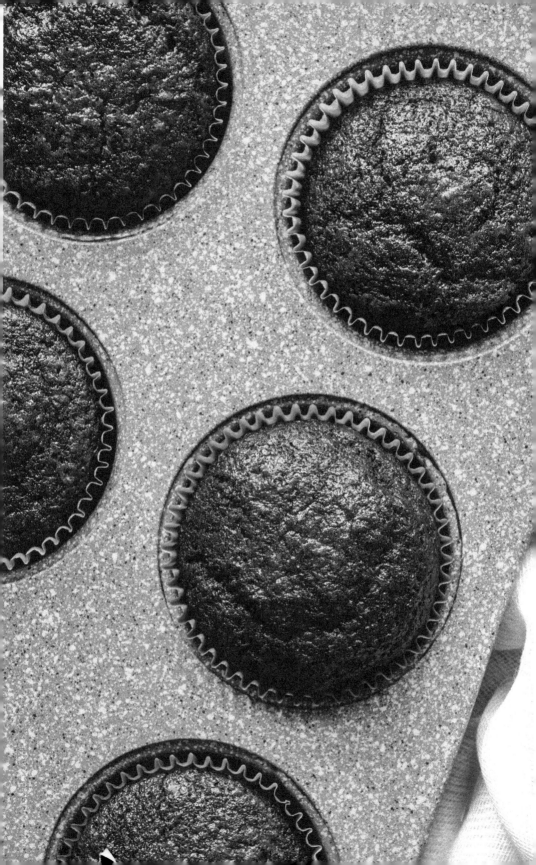

Chocolate Muffins

This recipe also makes a delicious chocolate cake for those special occasions.

INGREDIENTS

2 cups of grated pumpkin*
2 free range eggs
½ cup light tasting olive oil
4 tablespoons maple syrup**
1 teaspoon vanilla extract
¾ cup of good quality cocoa or cacao powder
1 teaspoon baking soda
2 teaspoons baking powder
¼ teaspoon salt
¼ cup coconut flour

INSTRUCTIONS

Preheat oven to 180°C.
Lightly beat the eggs and place in a large bowl with the pumpkin, maple syrup, vanilla and oil. Stir to combine.
Next, sift in the cacao, coconut flour, baking soda, baking powder and sea salt.
Stir gently until well combined.
Pour about ¼ -½ cup into muffin tins. You should get 8 good sized muffins from the mixture.
Bake until firm to touch (roughly 20 minutes).

*You can also try experimenting with beetroot or kumara.
** Any liquid sweetener will do for this recipe. They are also still delicious without any added sweetener.

Crowding in
the 'Good' Stuff

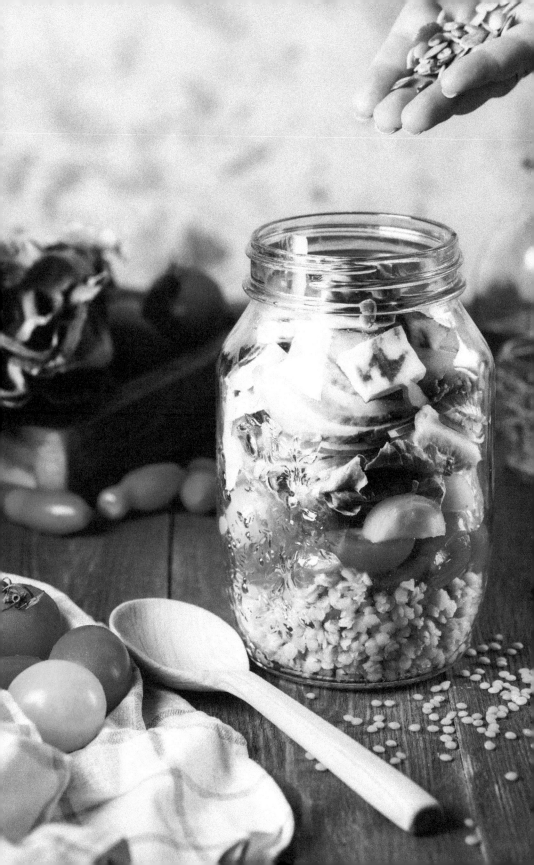

We all have our own personal, and usually quite long, lists of foods that we avoid because of this or that reason.

We're told by both the media and professionals that certain foods are harmful and we need to QUIT them, pronto.

Unfortunately, when you focus on quitting certain foods the same scenario often happens. When you tell someone they can't have something that they love, more often than not, they will begin to crave that food more. This will lead to despair, to eventually giving up and over indulging, which is followed by guilt and shame and the cycle continues. Too often, people are confusing healthy eating with "all or nothing", which ultimately leads to this cycle of restriction-deprivation-surrender then guilt. But it doesn't have to be this way!

What if, we looked at things a bit differently.
What if, instead of thinking of which foods you have to give up, you start to focus on what nourishing foods you can add in?

Crowding-in is a concept I use frequently in my practice. It simply means changing your focus to getting more nutrient-rich foods rather than putting your attention on cutting out the other foods.

The focus is on increasing foods that serve you so that eventually there is less room for the ones that don't. Even if the rest of your diet doesn't completely change – you're still going to get more nutrients and eating more healthy foods, and I believe that eventually you'll begin to change your taste buds and start to crave foods that nourish you.

Focus on the good and you'll attract more of the same. Your body and mind will thank you.

What does crowding-in look like?
It is about serving up an abundance of vegetables at dinner, adding spinach to your scrambled eggs, or drinking a glass of water before reaching for that sweet snack. It's about being creative and asking yourself: "How can I crowd-in more veggies with this meal?" or "What oil might be better for cooking?"

This approach, which focuses on taking small daily steps and increasing healthy food rather than avoiding indulgences creates a much more positive framework for implementing lasting change. It has been shown over and over again to lead to more lasting results with health goals.

When you add in wholesome nutrient-dense ingredients, your health is going to immediately benefit from the extra vitamins, minerals and antioxidants you're consuming, and it can be as simple as adding blueberries to your porridge!

Over the next chapters I'll be sharing with you tips and tricks for crowding-in more colourful vegetables, quality proteins and the healthiest of fats. While you're at it, why not crowd in a little self care as well!?

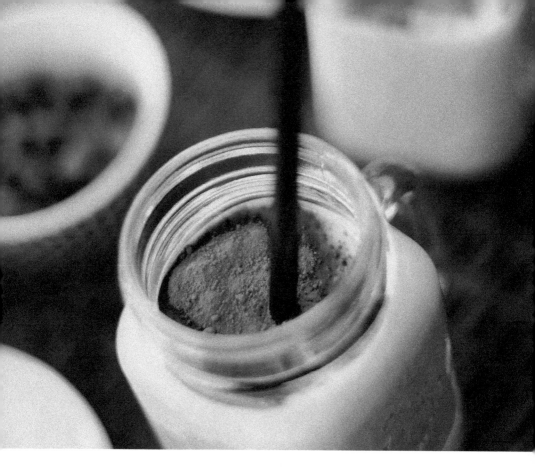

Chocolate Covered Berries Smoothie

Here is a great summer smoothie that crowds in heaps of the stuff your body loves!

INGREDIENTS

Serves 1

1 cup almond milk
½ cup frozen berries
1 tablespoon ground linseed
1 tablespoon chia seeds
1 tablespoon raw cacao powder
(or cocoa)
1 scoop of vanilla pea protein or your
favourite sweet protein powder.
¼ of an avocado

INSTRUCTIONS

Blend all of the ingredients in a
high-speed blender and enjoy!

INDULGE,
SIT BACK AND
ENJOY THE
GRATITUDE
FROM YOUR
BODY.

———

The Powerhouse *of Nutrition*

If there is one thing that EVERYONE would agree we need to get more of in our diets it's definitely fruit and vegetables.

There are debates over fat, sugar, protein, meat and many other things but when it comes to vegetables, everyone seems to get along.

Last chapter I introduced you to the nutritional concept of 'crowding in'. The idea that to lovingly nourish your body you should focus on getting more of the good stuff rather than dwelling on what you think you shouldn't have.

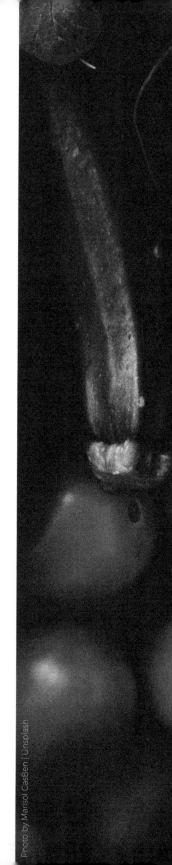

Photo by Marisol CasBen | Unsplash

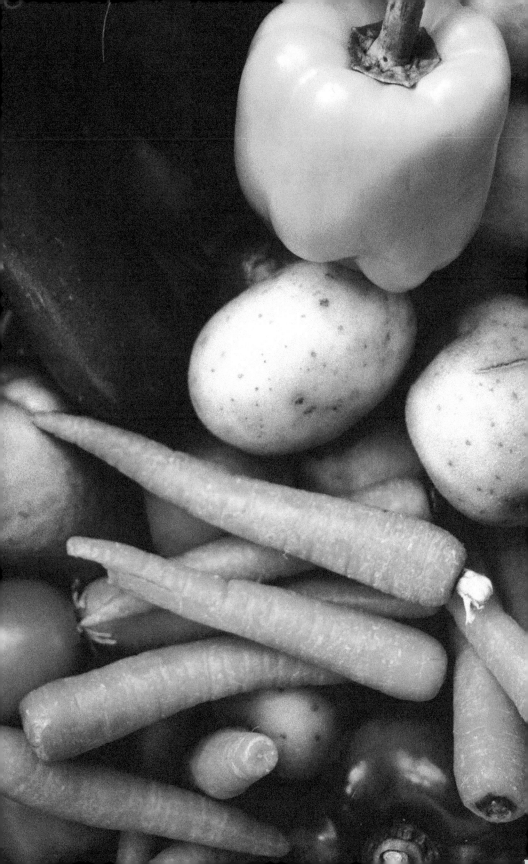

Veggies are nutrition packed powerhouses. They have an abundance of micro-nutrients that just make you feel amazing inside and out.

The more variety of vegetables you get each day the better you'll feel.

By crowding in more veggies, you can enjoy more energy, clearer skin, a healthier body, better concentration and overall fabulous feeling. Not only that but you're naturally crowding out other options that might make you feel less so.

Government dietary guidelines recommend at least 5 servings of fruit and vegetables a day. Five a day? Pfft that's so last year!

Ideally, all our plates will be made up of at least ½ veggies and in a perfect world you would be eating them in between meals as well. I'd love you all to be having a variety of bright colourful veggies a day, antioxidant-rich berries and seasonal fruit. Bring back the meat and three vege I say!

So, how do you fit in so many vegetables?
You don't need to live off salads! It's really not as daunting as it sounds and if you grow them yourself, or choose seasonal varieties, it doesn't

need to cost much either. Here are some common ways I crowd in these little gems each day.

Add to scrambles: I love eating eggs, nature's multi-vitamin, but why not give them a boost by adding some greens, mushrooms, tomatoes or capsicums.

Spirilize: If you haven't got a spiralizer – you need one! Kids love watching the curly courgette noodles come through the other end (ok I admit it, I love it too) and they make a great addition to your spaghetti bolognaise. When it comes to pasta, it's really the sauce that adds the flavour so why not add to your noodles some spirilized courgette or other veggies to boost nutrition and flavour.

Boost your rice: Curry is delicious with a bed of greens. Again, it's the curry itself that packs a flavour punch and the rice is really just a way to add some bulk. So, why not serve your curry on a bed of sautéed greens? Another alternative is to grate some cauliflower and lightly sautee then add to your rice.

Hide in stews, stews and curries: Finely chop some greens and tell the family it's fresh herbs – or better yet – add some fresh herbs as well!

Boost your snacks: There are some pretty amazing green snacks out there these days. Kale chips can be purchased from just about any health-minded store and are also really easy to make. Or simply make a dip with kimchi and coconut yogurt and enjoy with carrots, cucumber, capsicum or other dippers!

Use as a wrap or burger bun: I know, it doesn't sound nearly as exciting but trust me, once you try it, you'll love it. Even popular restaurants and take-away places now offer bun-less options.

Add them to smoothies: Smoothies are the ultimate place to get some veggies. If you really want to go incognito blend into your favourite chocolate smoothie with greens and no one will know. Spinach and silver beet have a fairly neutral tastes so are my top choices when it comes to covert smoothie action. Another trick I enjoy is freezing chopped courgette or cauliflower for smoothies. They make the smoothie creamy and cold without changing the flavour.

Making a berry smoothie? Why not add some red capsicum – it's adds to the vibrant colour and compliments the berries perfectly.

Summer Salad

There are so many ways to get more veggies in your diet. Start one step at a time, and use your imagination. Look at your current meals and ask yourself how you might be able to crowd in some colour. Here's one of my favourite veggie packed recipes. Enjoy!

INGREDIENTS

Serves 2

1 packet of smoked salmon
(feel free to omit if vegetarian)

5 strawberries

2 cups salad greens

1 courgette

1½ tablespoons balsamic vinegar

3 tablespoons olive oil (lemon infused olive oil is also nice)

Fresh thyme sprigs

INSTRUCTIONS

Drizzle a little bit of olive oil in a frying pan. Cut your courgette into small rounds and gently saute until just cooked. Set aside. Place the salad green in a bowl and top with the cooked courgette, strawberries and salmon. Drizzle with the vinegar and olive oil.

For a more concentrated flavour – drizzle with balsamic reduction (but you won't need as much!). Sprinkle the salads with fresh thyme.

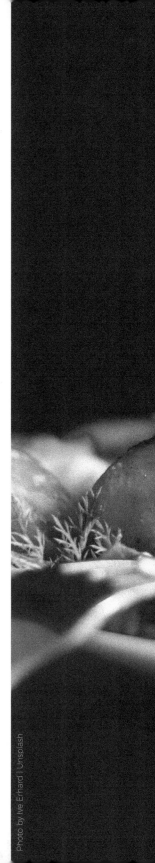

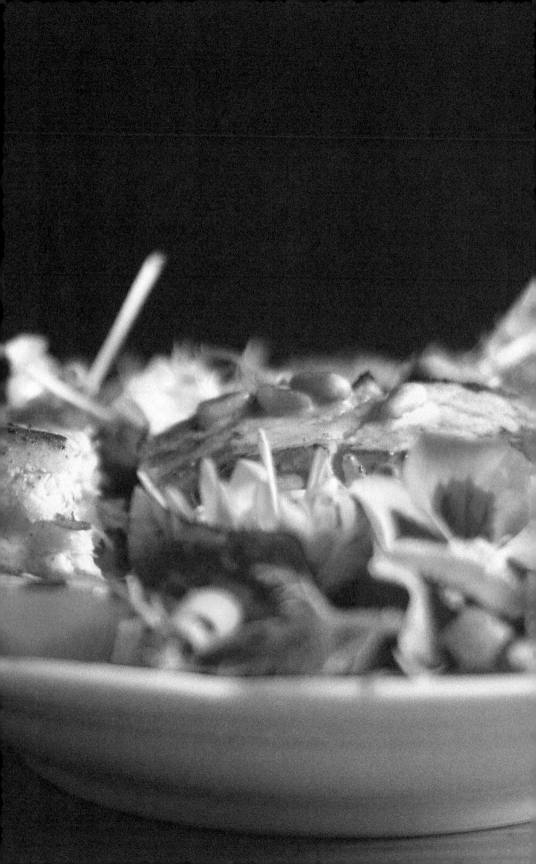

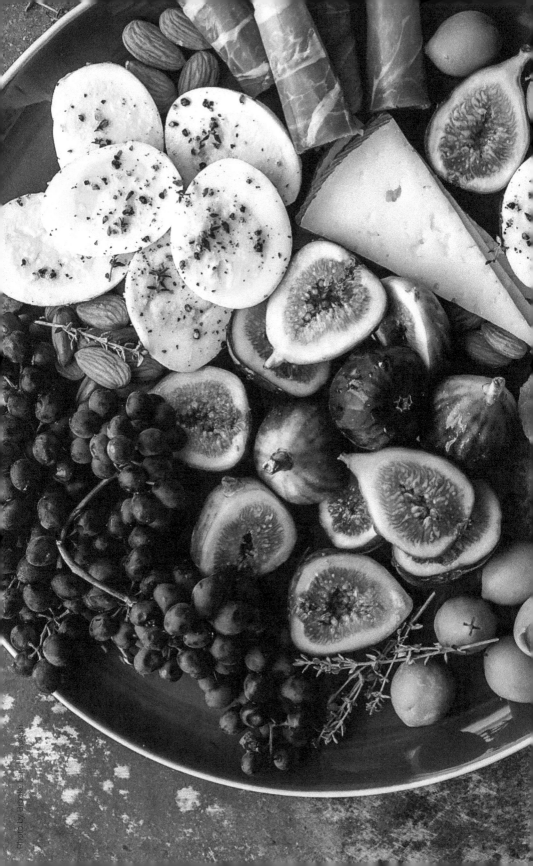

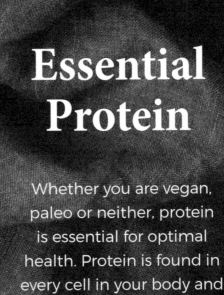

Essential Protein

Whether you are vegan, paleo or neither, protein is essential for optimal health. Protein is found in every cell in your body and plays a role in basic bodily functions – from walking to digesting food.

So far you have learnt how a focus on getting more of the good stuff rather than restriction. This is key when it comes to sustainable health.

We have looked at fruit and vegetables so far and we will begin to look at a variety of ways to crowd in more fibre, healthy fats, carbs and vitamins and minerals further on, but in this chapter I want to talk to you about protein – why we need it and where to get it.

Protein builds, repairs and maintains muscle tissue, can help maintain healthy skin and hair, is involved in the production of enzymes and hormones and can also support your immune system. It is referred to as an essential nutrient for a reason!

Protein helps to promote optimal levels of fullness so that you can feel more satisfied in-between meals. It also has a significant role in keeping your blood sugars balanced throughout your day helping prevent the highs and lows that can occur without.

When it comes to crowding-in, how much protein should we be consuming?

Ideally you are eating protein throughout the day, at both meals and snacks (if you need them). When it comes to how much, I usually stick to the palm-sized recommendation as a starting point. You may need more, or less, depending on your unique body. You'll find that because of the satiating ability of protein you may not get as hungry as often and your energy is more consistent. Having protein at lunch can also help prevent that dreaded afternoon-slump.

Eating a variety of different protein sources is important and will improve the likelihood of you getting a complete intake of the amino acids your body needs. This is especially true if you don't eat animal proteins.

If you eat animal protein, I suggest choosing ethically raised meats and fish. These may cost more but the importance is quality, not quantity when it comes to animal protein.

Great vegetarian sources of protein include nuts, seeds (such as chia seeds, sunflower, pumpkin and sesame), legumes and eggs.

There are also some fabulous protein powders available here in New Zealand (and worldwide) that are perfect for smoothies as well as gluten free baking. For those who consume dairy products, whey is another great option.

Play around with different protein sources and pay attention to your hunger and energy levels when you crowd them in.

———

YOU ARE YOUR
OWN GURU,
LISTEN CLOSELY
AND YOUR BODY
WILL GIVE YOU
THE ANSWERS.

Love Balls

INGREDIENTS

½ cup sunflower seeds

½ cup pumpkin seeds

½ cup sesame seeds

½ cup sesame seed butter (Tahini)

½ cup 85% dark chocolate, chopped

½ cup organic dried cranberries or cherries

2 tablespoons maple syrup

INSTRUCTIONS

Process the seeds in a food processor until well chopped and fine.

Add the chocolate and cranberries and pulse a few times until chopped. Then add these and all the remaining ingredients to a bowl. Shape into walnut sized balls.

If the mixture is too sticky to roll into balls – place in the fridge until the mixture hardens a little bit. Alternatively, you could press into a baking paper lined slice tray and cut these into slices.

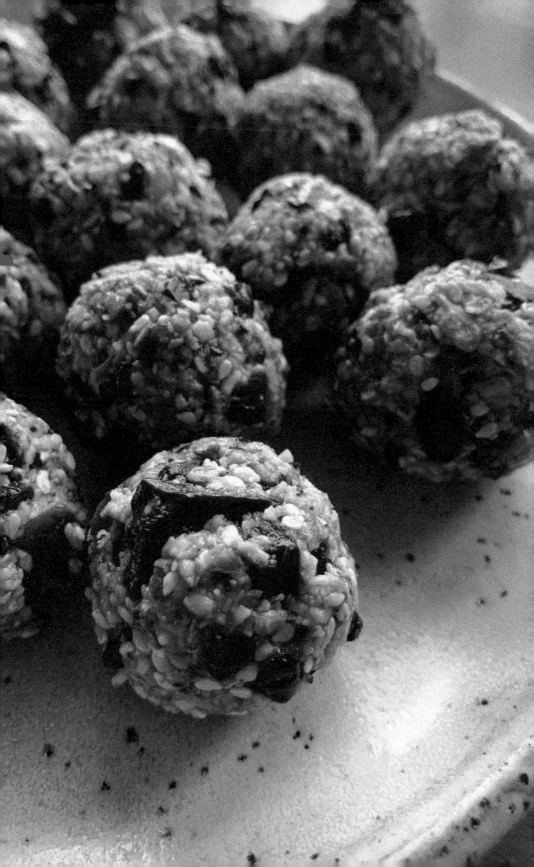

Fats
that Fuel

I can vividly remember being a young girl on a diet happily munching on lollies to my heart's content – because they were fat-free.

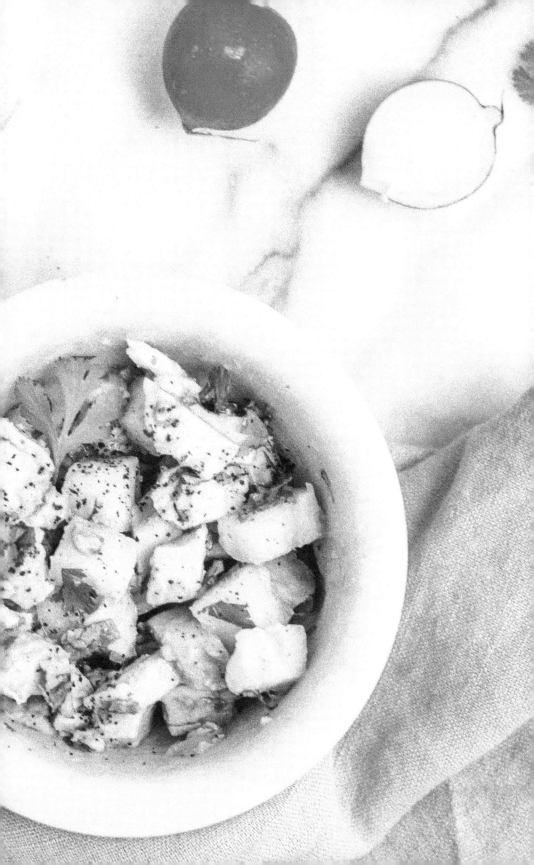

Yes! There are fats that your body needs and that you should be crowding-in daily.

Times have certainly changed, and while I don't believe that sugar needs to be our next scapegoat, it's important to realise that fat is back, and it is super important for healthy bodies.

Personally, I think a lot of the fat fears stem from an increase in processed foods and take-aways. Those types of fats are an entirely different story than the ones that nature produces. People began consuming unimaginable quantities of heavily processed fats in various forms, and like most things, too much of any food can lead to concerns.

Meanwhile, there are some fats that your body needs and that you should consider crowding-in to your daily routine. These fats are great for your brain, hair, nails, skin and for your overall health. They are vital to every single cell in your body as well as being crucial for the absorption of vitamins A, D, E and K.

There are several different types of fats available:

Saturated Fat: Mainly from animal sources such as meat and butter, but also in coconut oil (though it's a medium-chain fatty acid).

Trans fats: While they occur naturally in some foods in small amounts they are more commonly seen in highly processed foods.

Monounsaturated fats: Such as olive oil, sesame oil and safflower oil.

Polyunsaturated Fats: Soy oil, corn oil and sunflower oil are some examples.

Omega 3: These are also polyunsaturated fats but are so important I've given them their own category. These include fats from fatty fish and some plants such as flaxseed and chia seeds.

It can all get a bit confusing at times, and so like most things when it comes to nutrition, I like to say – KEEP IT SIMPLE.

In general, when it comes to swapping out for better and best choices I like to stick to the ones that are made with the least amount of processing. Cold pressed oils, moderate amounts of animal fats, nuts seeds and avocados. For those who can tolerate dairy, I suggest full fat dairy, and cheese on occasion rather than the low-fat varieties. Start with all this and you're doing your body a wealth of good.

1. https://authoritynutrition.com/13-benefits-of-fish-oil/

Which fats do I choose most often?
My cupboards are never without olive oil, I think it's my Mediterranean ancestry!

For cooking, I love to use light tasting olive oil for everything from sautéing to roasting. Contrary to popular belief, these types are cooking methods are perfectly fine for olive oil!

I also love avocado oil, macadamia oil and sesame oil – it depends on what I'm having.

For drizzling and dressings and smoothies: Hemp oil, a robust olive oil, flax oil, avocado oil and macadamia oil are all my go-to, depending what's on hand.

I also recommend everyone take a good fish oil supplement if you do not consume fatty fish a minimum of twice per week. [1]

How much fat should you be consuming? It really depends on the individual but ultimately, just because fat is important doesn't mean you should have bucket loads of the stuff. A healthy diet is all about balance, variety and moderation, and like most things, with fats I suggest you get a variety from both plants and animals and to pair them up with an abundance of fruits, vegetables and quality proteins.

A HEALTHY OUTSIDE, STARTS FROM THE INSIDE.

RICHARD URICH

———————

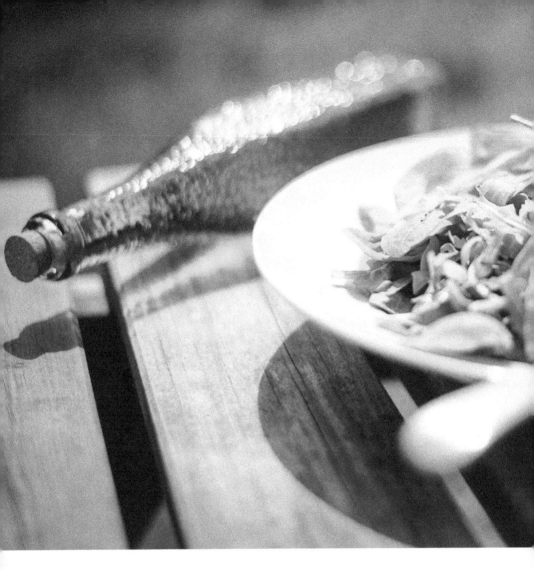

Super Speedy Salad Dressing

INGREDIENTS

½ cup olive oil

2 tablespoons balsamic or
cider vinegar

2 tablespoons lemon juice

1 pinch of salt

1 tsp Dijon mustard

INSTRUCTIONS

Place all the ingredients in a small
jar and give a good shake. Double up
the recipe and keep in the fridge for
quick and easy salads.

This is also delicious drizzled over
roasted veggies!

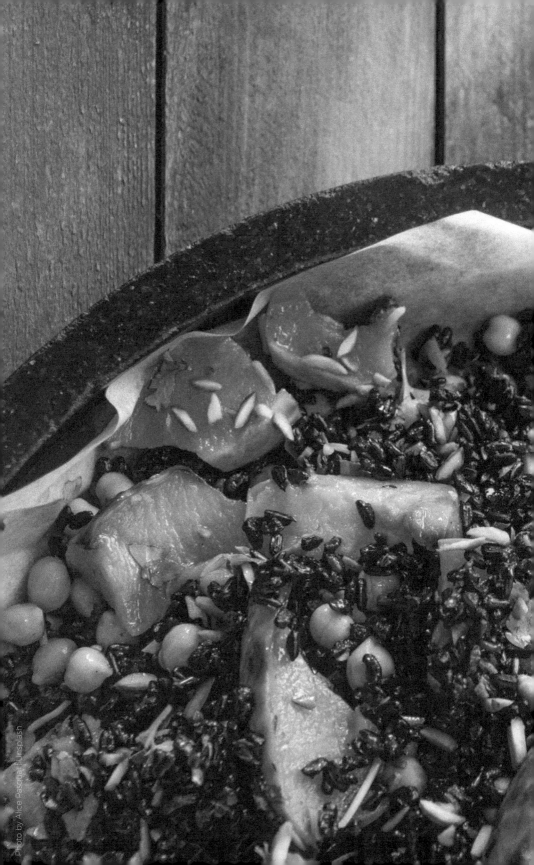

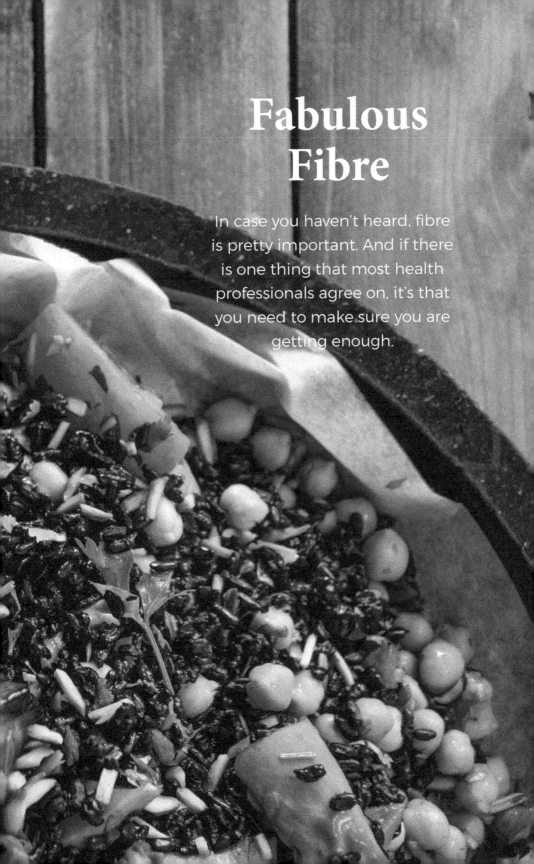

Fabulous Fibre

In case you haven't heard, fibre is pretty important. And if there is one thing that most health professionals agree on, it's that you need to make sure you are getting enough.

So what's with fibre?
Why is it so important?
And how do you get more of it?

Let's start by looking at the what –
basically, there are two main types
of fibre and that is based on their
solubility in water.

It's no surprise then that they are
referred to as soluble and insoluble
fibre.

Within that, there are many different
kinds as well as some overlapping
amongst the two.

So why should you keep tabs on the
amount of fibre you're consuming?
If you're often hungry some types of
fibre can help by keeping you fuller
for longer.

Add in some healthy fats and protein
and you've got a winning combo for
satiety. Try adding some psyllium or
flax seeds to your porridge or simply
put a teaspoons or two of chia seeds
into your smoothie to reap
the benefits.

Another way that fibre can help
support your body and overall
health is by feeding the beneficial
bacteria in the gut. A healthy
digestive system is a happy digestive
system. Your gut is essentially the
hub of the wheel and by keeping
it well populated with beneficial
bacteria and feeding the critters
regularly you can benefit from blood
sugar regulation, immune support
and brain function.

Fibre has been shown to help regulate
blood sugar in general if your meal
is slightly more carb-loaded and has
been beneficial in reducing total
cholesterol levels.

Ultimately in all these cases, the
type of fibre is important and
so the bottom line is to strive to
get a variety of different sources
throughout your day.

Avocados are a good source of fibre and with those great fats can keep you fuller for longer.

My first go-to sources for fibre are fruits and vegetables. Aiming to have five plus servings a day of veggies plus a couple servings of fruit is sure to give you a good variety of healthy fibre as well as an abundance of vitamins and minerals. Start there!

Some seeds are very rich sources especially chia seeds and flax seeds.

Whole grains can be a great source of dietary fibre though less refined is best. My favourite sources include oats, farro bread and buckwheat.

If you're able to digest them effectively, beans and legumes can also be a great source of fibre. Lentils, chickpeas, beans of all sorts can be added to stews, sauces and salads as a great addition to a healthy diet.

If all you did was increase your veggies and enjoy a variety of fruits and seeds you'd be making great big steps in the right direction.

Your gut and your overall health will thank you!

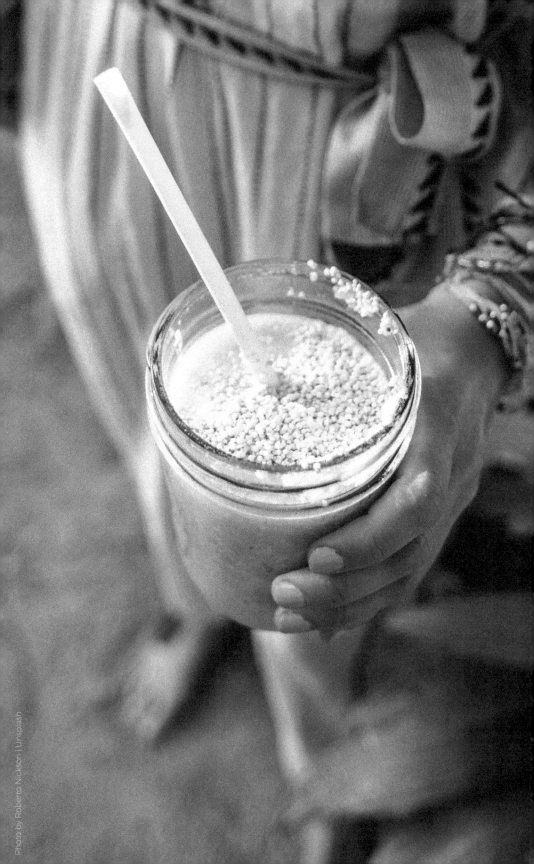

Good Green Smoothie

INGREDIENTS

1 cup unsweetened coconut or almond milk

1 teaspoon pure vanilla extract

1 small green banana (I know it looks like it's not ready – but is a good source of resistant starch).

¼ avocado

½ teaspoon cardamom powder

1 tablespoon chia seeds

1 handful of spinach

1 scoop vanilla protein powder (optional)

INSTRUCTIONS

Blend with ice and enjoy.

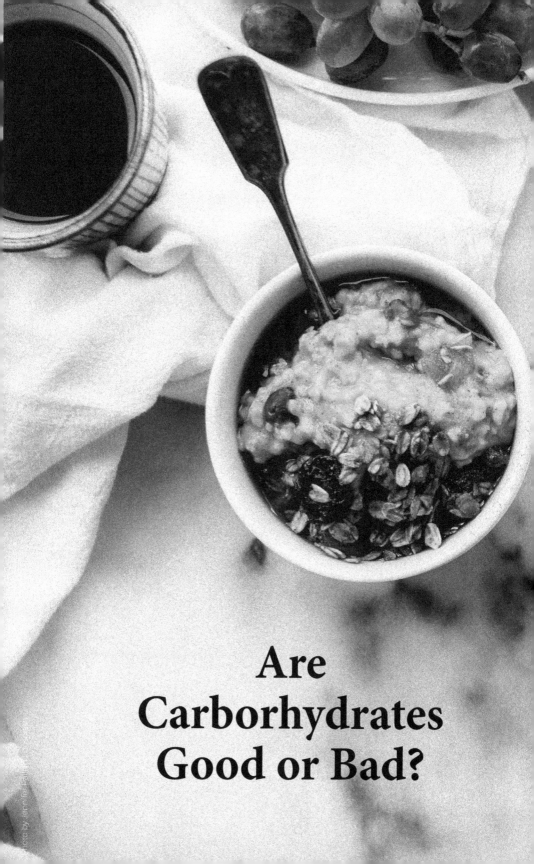

Are Carborhydrates Good or Bad?

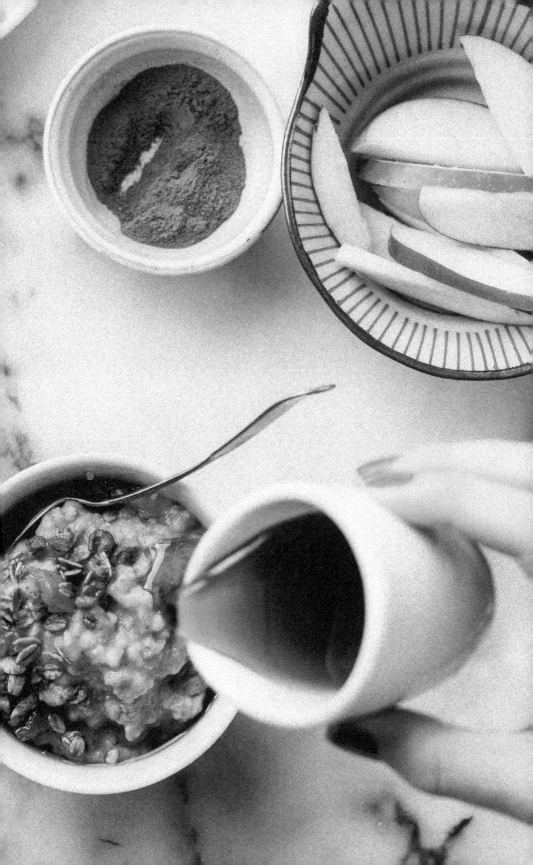

There's a lot of debate in the nutrition world when it comes to carbs. Everywhere you look carbs are branded as either good or bad and if people have weight loss goals they are often, unnecessarily, told to avoid them.

First, what are carbs? Are they just potatoes, bread and rice?

Carborhydrates (carbs) are found in so many foods including dairy products, fruit, vegetables, grains, nuts, legumes, seeds and sugary foods and sweets.

They are made up of three components: FIBRE, STARCH and SUGAR

Fibre and starch are complex carbs, while sugar is a simple carb. When it comes to carbs, they all have a place in your diet but nutrient-wise, the more complex the carb is, the more nutrients it contains.

Complex carbs have a variety of nutrients depending on the food and more fibre which can fill you up for longer. These include fruit, vegetables, legumes, whole grains and seeds. Almost all centenarians (those who live past 100) have some level of complex carbohydrate rich foods in their diets.

Simple carbs are sugars. They burn quickly and can leave you hungry and wanting more. But are they bad? Ultimately, no food is bad or good, it's the dose that matters, but they do not have as many of the nutrients that your body needs and so I'd classify them as 'soul foods' – think birthday cake or fish and chips on a Friday.

How many carbs a person needs depends on a couple of things. Their body's ability to process them and the amount of energy that they burn in a typical day. The more active you are, the more energy you'll burn

So what's the deal with carbs, are they the big bad wolf we're led to believe they are?

and complex carbs can definitely be helpful. Carbs are not classified as essential but they can certainly be beneficial… and tasty! Veggies and fruit are wonderful sources of nutrient dense carbs.

Fact is, there are some people who metabolise carbs better than others depending on everything from genetics to activity levels and so that's why it is so important to work out what works for you rather than just listen to what has worked for someone else.

If too many carbs leave you hungry, tired and grumpy, try having less or swapping out for more complex carbs to see if that makes a difference in your energy or hunger. If not, maybe reducing them will help.

All in all, try to avoid looking at carbs as simply 'carbs' and try to see all the good stuff they can contain as well. Carbs, like all foods, are not black and white and to avoid them completely if they make you feel great, is totally unnecessary.

Experiment by swapping out your carbs and listen to what your body tells you.

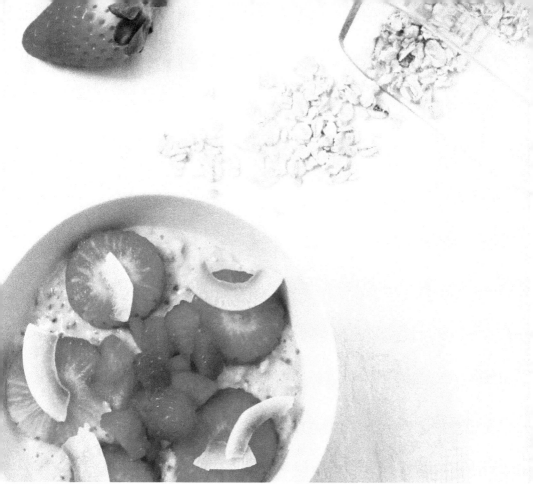

Summertime Oats

This cold version of porridge is just as filling
and comforting in the Summer months.

½ ripe banana mashed
1 teaspoon olive oil
1 tablespoon natural peanut butter
or almond butter
½ cup rolled oats
1 teaspoon chia seeds
1 cup almond milk or coconut milk
1 teaspoon ground cinnamon
1 scoop of your favourite protein
powder (optional – I recommend
Nuzest Vanilla Clean Lean Pea
Protein)

Mix all the ingredients in a medium
sized jar. Leave in the fridge overnight
and enjoy in the morning with your
favourite toppings. Some ideas
include berries, more sliced banana,
sliced apples, plain yogurt or all of the
above!

KEEP IT
SIMPLE, SHOW
YOUR BODY
THE LOVE IT
LONGS FOR
AND CONTINUE
TO PRACTICE
GRATITUDE, AND
YOUR BODY
WILL LOVE YOU
BACK.

———

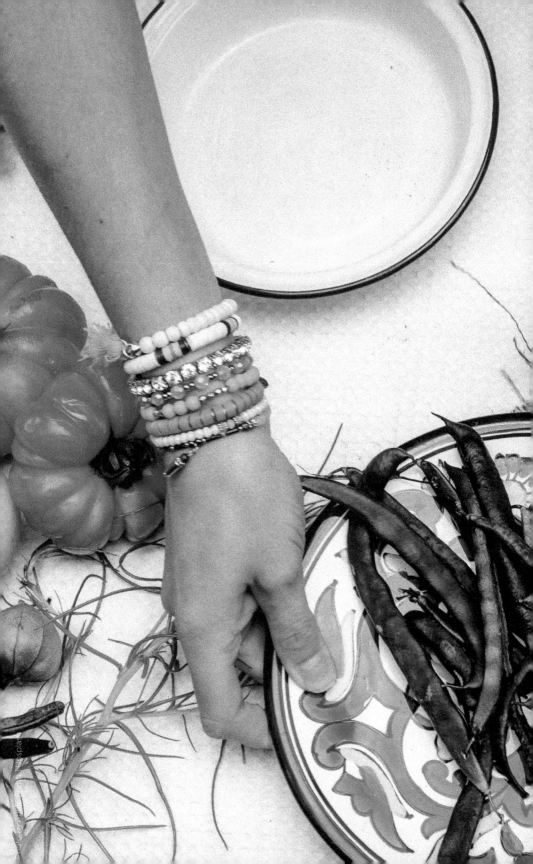

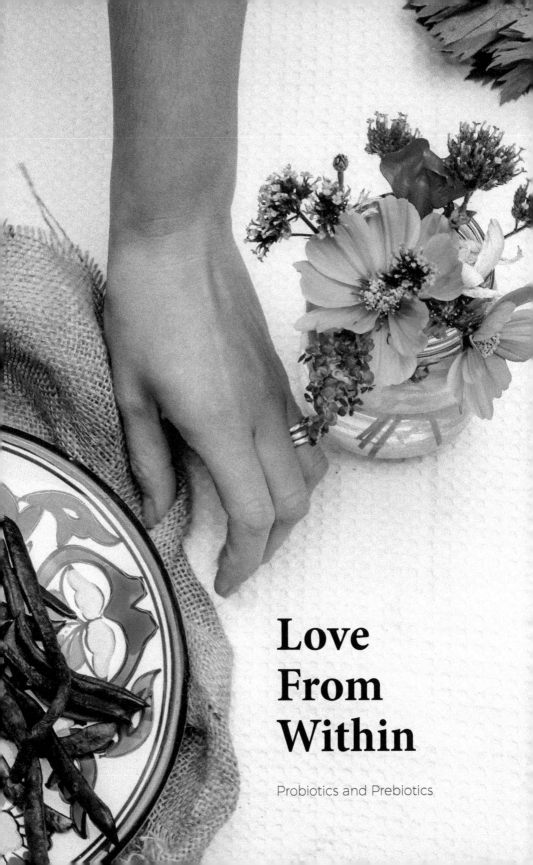

Love
From
Within

Probiotics and Prebiotics

You've crowded-in veggies, protein, healthy fats, carbs and fibre – now let's crowd in all those amazing micro-organisms that populate and feed your gut.

When I say THE GUT I'm essentially referring to the whole of our digestive system. It starts in the mouth and ends, well, you know where it ends! The gut's main roles are to absorb nutrients and get rid of the things that shouldn't be in our body.

If we were a wheel, our gut would be the hub. 80% of our immune system resides there and 90% of serotonin is created within it. Ultimately, if your gut isn't happy, you are not happy!

What do you need for a healthy gut?
Essentially, three things; a healthy immune system, an intact lining and a good balance of bacteria. I want to focus on the latter.

Did you know, that you have more bacteria in your body than there are human cells?
Overall we all have a couple of kilos of thousands of different strains of bacteria in our bodies at any given time. Diversity is important and the

complexity of that diversity is a result of different factors from food to birth to the amount of stress in our lives.

Good bacteria is important for gut health and are like tourists coming and going from your digestive system resort. With that in mind, it is important to continue to repopulate your gut bacteria through bacteria with a variety of natural foods and stress reduction food and lifestyle choices.

Are supplements necessary?

Perhaps in some cases, if you have been through a round of medications or a great deal of stress, but in most cases, I like to start people off with food first. By incorporating probiotic rich foods as well as pre-biotic foods into your everyday diet, you're doing your body (and brain) an abundance of good.

In a nutshell – probiotics are the good bacteria that your body needs and prebiotics are fibres that your body cannot digest, and serve as food for probiotics.

Luckily for us, there is a range of delicious probiotic and prebiotic rich foods that you can crowd into your diet.

Probiotic foods are the fermented goodies including (but not limited to):
Saurkraut
Kefir
Yogurt
Kānga pirau
Kimchi
Kombucha

Prebiotics are also abundant in the foods we eat!
Legumes, beans and peas
Oats
Bananas
Berries
Garlic
Leeks
Onions

By managing stress (like with the techniques shared by AwesoME Inc®) and crowding in fibre-rich vegetables as often as possible, plus adding 1-2 different fermented foods to your diet each day, you're well on your way to keeping your gut great.

Gut health doesn't have to be complicated or extreme, in fact stress – whether it be related to life or food – has just as severe an effect on the overall health of your digestive system.

Probiotic Guacamole

This dip is perfect with corn chips or chopped veggies and it's packed with both prebiotics and probiotics to boot!

Serves 2

1 ripe avocado

1 tablespoon lime or lemon juice

1 tablespoon lime coconut water kefir (or more lime juice)

1 heaped tablespoon of plain sauerkraut (or kimchi for a spicier flavour)

1 tablespoon chopped fresh coriander

1 clove of garlic, chopped

INSTRUCTIONS

Blend all the ingredients in a blender until smooth and creamy. Serve straight away.

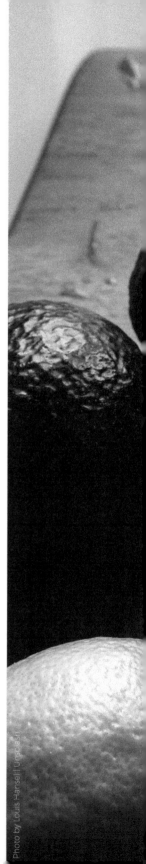

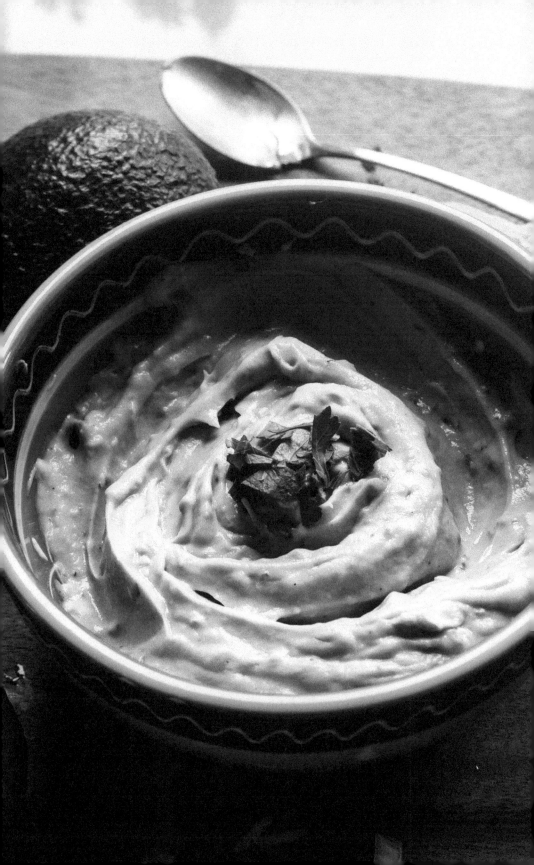

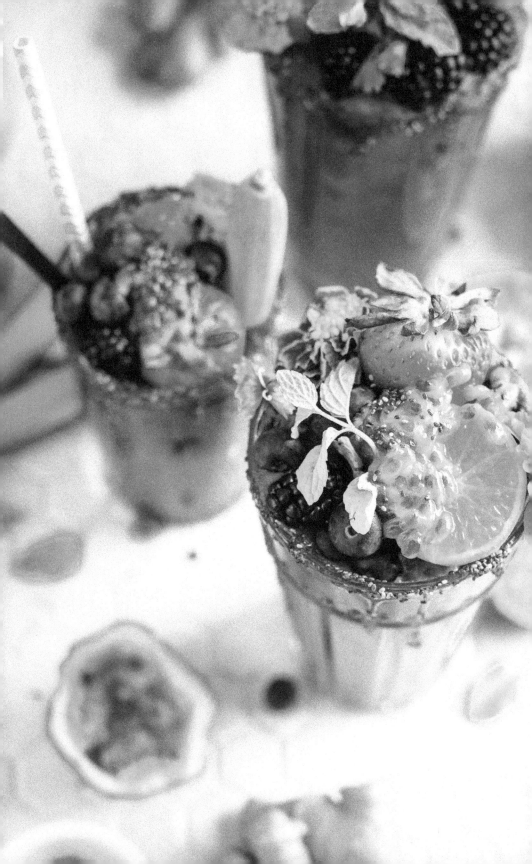

Be Mindful of
the Little Guys

Macronutrients

The foundation of Gentle Nutrition is understanding that your body needs certain nutrients to function optimally, but it is also about being able to balance foods that may not be so nutrient dense – without guilt, shame or anxiety.

We've looked at how to crowd in our essential macronutrients; protein and fat. We've bulked up on fibre and slow burning carbs and kept our bellies happy with probiotics. But what about the other little guys, those nutrients that are so small yet so vital to human health?

Micronutrients are the vitamins and minerals that your body needs to keep you feeling happy and healthy.

Unlike macronutrients you only need a teeny tiny amount to maintain good health and yet despite that, we find ourselves frequently deficient.

There are fat-soluble vitamins such as vitamins A, D, E and K. and water soluble vitamins including the B vitamins and vitamin C. There are also minerals such as magnesium, iron, calcium and potassium. All of which are needed to keep you feeling your best.

Deficiencies can have lasting effects on the health of both children and adults and so it's important to pay attention to your body and its warning signals when you're not feeling your best.

Governments have recognised the importance of these nutrients and created synthetic supplementation for everything from milk to cereals to orange juice. But are these synthetic vitamins really providing your body with the little guys you need?

In most cases, nutrients from whole foods should be your first choice. Whether these be plant based supplements or making sure to get a balanced diet with plenty of colourful vegetables and a variety of protein, fat and carb sources.

Some of my favourite nutrient-dense foods include:

KALE: Jam-packed with an abundance of vitamin C, vitamin A, vitamin K1 and vitamins B6, potassium, calcium, magnesium, copper and manganese! Plus there's plenty of fibre as well.

Micronutrients are essential for good health, and micronutrient deficiencies can cause serious health problems.

GARLIC: Tastes amazing and is also full of vitamins C, B1 and B6, calcium, potassium, copper, manganese and selenium.

SHELL-FISH: Clams are one of the best sources of B12 on the planet as well as vitamins C, B-vitamins, potassium, selenium and iron. Oysters also have an abundance of nutrients including zinc.

POTATOES: Surprised? Potatoes actually have a little bit of almost every nutrient you need as well as being incredibly satiating. If you cool potatoes and then reheat, or eat cold the next day, you've also got a powerful source of resistant starch.

EGGS: I like to refer to eggs as nature's multi-vitamin and most of the vitamins are found in the yolk. They also have healthy fats and proteins and are cheap, versatile and taste amazing.

There are so many nutrient-abundant natural foods being grown and raised here in New Zealand but sometimes a good multi-vitamin can be an insurance policy to fill any gaps.

When looking for a multi-vitamin there are a few things you should be aware of when reading the label:

Check that your supplement uses a ready to use folate rather than synthetic folic acid. Many of us can't metabolise synthetic folic acid. It is best to check that it contains natural folate altogether.

I also prefer natural sources of calcium from algae (if vegan/vegetarian) or natural dairy based sources rather than the lab-produced calcium citrate, carbonate and phosphate used in common multi-vitamins.

When it comes to B-12 (which is essential for brain health and a common deficiency in vegans and vegetarians) you want to look for a form that is already pre-converted and usable by your body. Most supplements use the common cyanocobalamin which is fine if your diet is perfect, stress is non existent and toxins don't exist. For the rest of us, methylcobalamin is the one you want to look for, it's already converted for you so your body can use it more efficiently.

Same with vitamin A, beta carotene can be difficult too for the body to convert in most cases and so look for a pre-formed retinyl palmitate instead.

There are some great companies out there that are using these more easily absorbed sources of vitamins and minerals.

As a general guideline, always choose food first but sometimes a quality food-based supplement or something equally as good is a healthy addition to your diet.

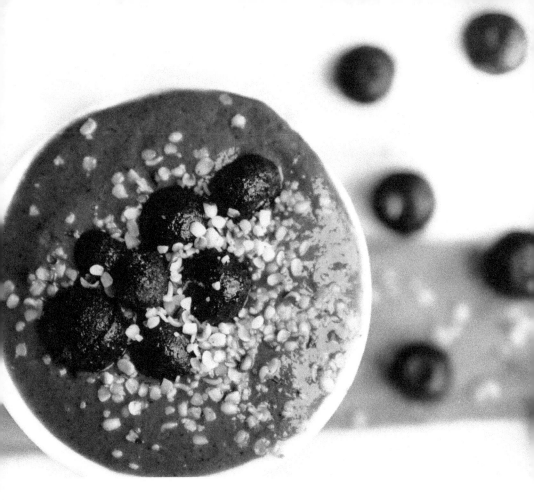

Kale, Blueberry
& Cream Smoothie

1 cup frozen blueberries

1 cup coconut milk

1 tablespoon ground linseeds

1 handful of kale (discard the stems)

1 splash of vanilla extract

1 pinch of cinnamon

1 tablespoon raw honey or a
drop of stevia

INSTRUCTIONS

Combine in a high speed blender
and enjoy.

Soul Food

This next chapter in our series of foods to crowd-in for health might surprise you, but I believe they are essential.

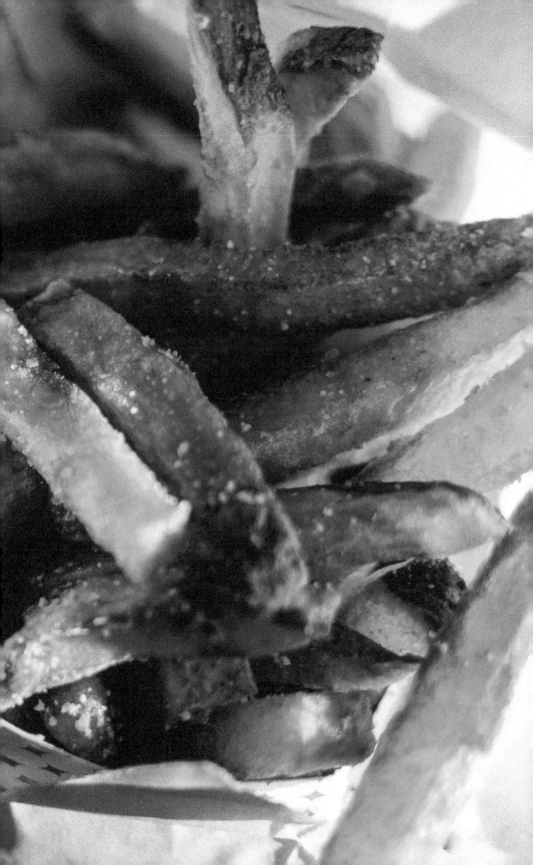

Soul foods nourish your heart and spirit and by doing so also nourish your physical body as well.

By soul foods, I mean those foods that may not necessarily be health approved but that make your soul sing. These are the chocolate cakes on your child's birthday, the fish and chips with your family on the beach or a decadent slice at a local café with your best friends.

What constitutes soul food for one person may differ from others but ultimately it is those foods commonly referred to as 'treats' in the sense that they just plain make you happy.

Contrary to popular belief there is no one food that will heal or harm, it is the dose that matters. Even too much kale could make you sick!

So why do I advocate including these foods in your lives?
Because when you label them as poison, toxic, bad, naughty or whatever other names you give them, and then restrict them, it ultimately leaves you wanting more anyway. Cravings are simply a result of deprivation.

Just imagine that I told you that starting tomorrow, you could never have your favourite food again. I don't know about you, but I know I'd be going out and overdoing it on that food as soon as possible.

Demonising food only puts it on a pedestal and gives it far too much power.

enjoyable treat turns into a week of indulgence, guilt and shame.

Surely it would be more beneficial to just eat it, enjoy it, be grateful and move on?

So how do we crowd in soul foods without worrying about it turning to a week-long binge?
I admit that this takes some time for some but by engaging in some of the following steps you're heading in the right direction.

Practice acceptance of all foods.
Knowing you can have a particular food if you want it creates abundance. Scarcity simply drives up the need while abundance makes you feel safe and comfortable in knowing that you can enjoy this food when the time comes. For me, this meant my cravings disappearing and getting much more enjoyment out of food. In between, eat a variety of nutrient dense foods that your body needs and enjoy the times when an opportunity to have some soul food pops up.

Make quality matter.
Just like for the French - the quality of your indulgences is important. Why waste an enjoyable bit of soul food on cheap junk (unless you LOVE cheap junk). If you want chocolate – get the best you can buy.

Many European cultures and even those hot spot blue zones (where people live well into their hundreds) engage in the food as a celebration. For the French, in particular, food is a pleasure and food quality is imperative. When enjoying bread, chocolate, or whatever soul food you want to include, make sure that it is made with quality ingredients, it is satisfying and pleasurable, and the experience is that of gratitude.
That is the joy of eating many of us are missing.

Instead, if you deprive, deprive, deprive until you cave, well we all know what happens then. You will feel like you blew it, so you might as well keep going! A delicious

LIFE IS JUST
TOO SHORT AND
FOOD IS FAR TOO
ENJOYABLE!

———

Love bread? Grab something fresh and delicious. You'll find yourself far more satisfied in the long run and less likely to over do it.

Start with a standard serving size or take yourself out to a café or restaurant.
This just helps to break the hypnosis of eating and gives you a chance to slow down and truly enjoy it.

Make sure you want it.
When was the last time you actually checked in to ask yourself if you genuinely want a certain food? Most people tend to grab and go with food and eat unconsciously –so by pressing pause you're enabling yourself to check in, Assess whether you actually feel like this treat or whether you're simply grabbing it because it's there. Check in with what I call 'The 4 Really Rule' – stop, check in and ask yourself if you "really, really, really, really" want it. If the answer is yes, proceed to the next two steps.

Eat mindfully.
So you've got an opportunity to eat some soul food, yay, now enjoy it! We call ourselves foodies and yet we can eat entire meals in minutes. If you can take the time to truly experience the complex flavours, aromas and textures of your favourite foods the experience is going to go a lot further. Think of it like a fine wine – make it an experience and enjoy each bite slowly engaging all of your senses.

Eat gratefully.
This is so important! If you're eating a food, that you may have once branded as bad, I want you to work towards changing your thinking knowing that no one food will harm you. Instead of anxiety or guilt – truly take a moment to enjoy what you're eating. Savour it and express sincere gratitude that you get to enjoy such an amazing food, know you can have it again, celebrate each experience and move on. Compassion is key.

My mission as a nutrition coach is to help people achieve their health goals without having to give up their favourite foods.

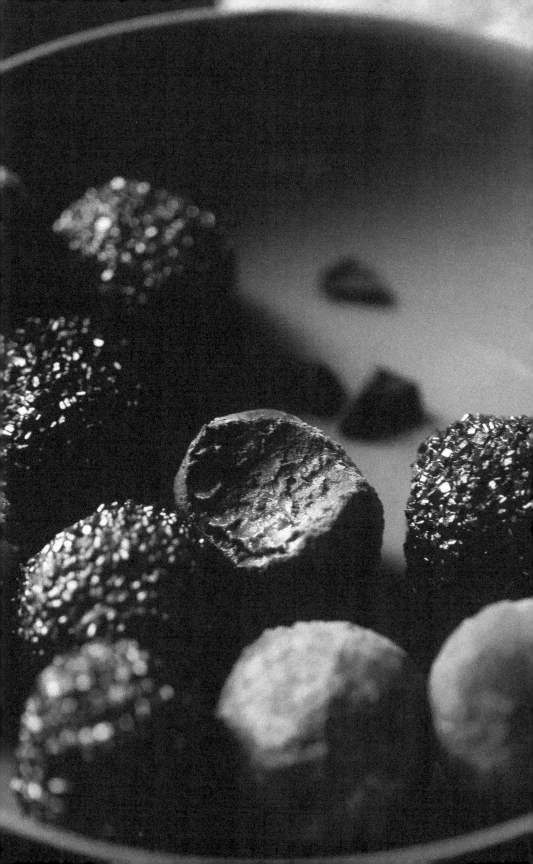

Decadent Dark Chocolate Truffles

These truffles will nourish the heart AND body. Enjoy!

INGREDIENTS

6 tablespoons smooth cashew butter

2 tablespoons coconut oil, melted

4 tablespoons cacao powder

2 tablespoons coconut nectar or maple syrup

1/4 teaspoon sea salt

1 teaspoon vanilla extract

150 grams 70-85% dark chocolate

INSTRUCTIONS

Mix all the ingredients together except for the chocolate. Pour into mini muffin moulds or other suitable moulds. Place in the freezer to harden.

Meanwhile, melt the dark chocolate over a double boiler. Once the mixture in the freezer is hard. Remove from the moulds and use a fork to dip each one into the melted chocolate. Place on a baking paper lined board of some sort and then return to the freezer to harden.

Drink Up!

When talking about nourishing your body, it's important that you don't forget hydration! There is so much confusion when it comes to how much and what that sometimes it can be overwhelming.

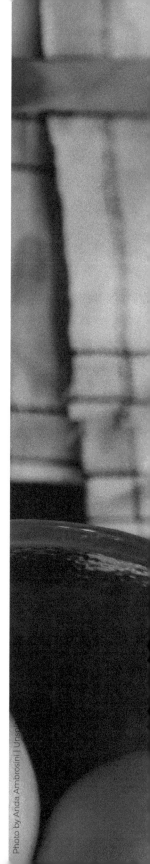

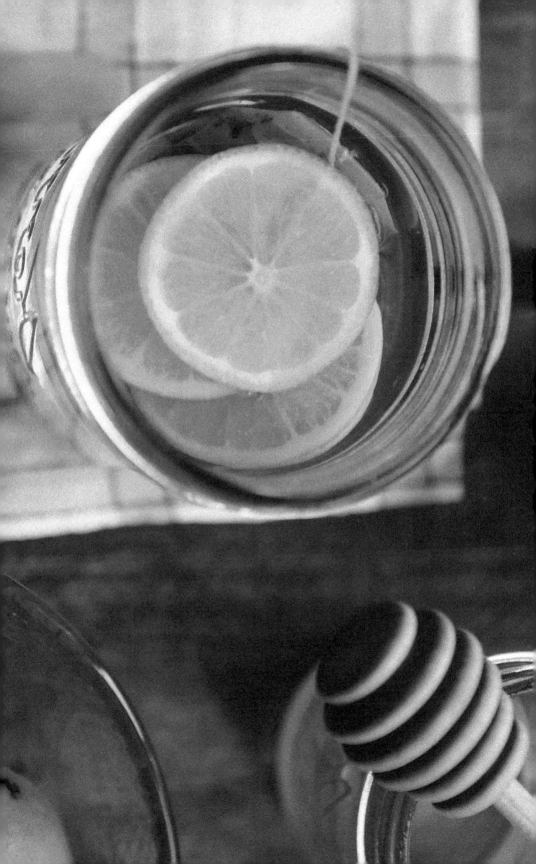

Should you drink eight glasses of water a day? Is coffee bad for you? What milk should you be drinking, if any? What if you don't like the taste of water? Can alcohol be part of a healthy diet?

Right, so first, when it comes to water it truly is imperative that you drink it! As a human you are over 60% water. Your body uses water in all its cells, organs, and tissues to help regulate its temperature and maintain other bodily functions. Because your body loses water just from living, it's important to rehydrate.

Do you need eight glasses a day?

Not necessarily. The amount of water you need depends on a variety of factors, including the climate you live in, how physically active you are, and whether you're experiencing an illness or have any other health concerns. I always think back to my distant ancestors and think – what would they do? Would they be counting out their eight glasses per day? Or would they be responding to their body's physical signs of dehydration or thirst?

If it's hot out, and you're sweating – you tend to become thirstier if you're exercising or moving your body a lot. It's also really easy to see from your urine whether you're dehydrated or not and adjust your water levels accordingly. Your urine should be a light yellow to clear colour – getting lighter as the day goes on.

You don't just have to hydrate with water though! There are lots of beverages that are equally as hydrating including herbal teas, juice, smoothies, etc. If you don't like the taste of water try adding a splash of juice, or lemon sweetened stevia. Kombucha is a fermented beverage that is low in sugar and tastes great too.

What about coffee?

Coffee gets a bad rep in the world of nutrition however a lot of it, if not most of it, is not accurate. As long as you're not feeling anxious or getting an upset tummy, shakes or other adverse effects then go ahead – grab that cuppa!

Surprisingly, when studies were done, it was found that coffee is also hydrating, which would explain why my husband manages to survive with very little water but heaps of coffee (but I'm not recommending you do that!).

There are lots of beverages that are equally as hydrating as water, including herbal teas, juice and smoothies.

What about milk?

Many of my clients want to know whether you should drink full fat, trim or any at all. Again I ask you to think back – would your great-grandmother have removed all that rich cream from her milk before drinking? When you remove the fat from milk, through homogenizing and pasteurizing, the vital nutrients are also removed, which is why milk is then fortified with synthetic vitamins and minerals. Natural is way more satisfying so don't shy away from adding it to your favourite cuppa or muesli.

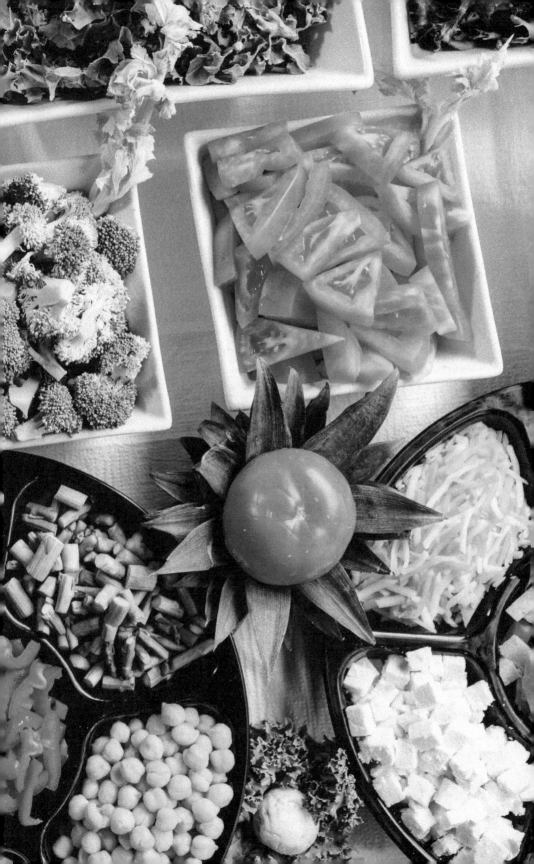

The Best 'Diet'
in the World

If you have a long history of
dieting this chapter is for you!

If you are like me you've probably tried all the diets! In the 80s, when I started, it was all about Weight Watchers, Richard Simmons and Jenny Craig. Atkins came later then Mediterranean, Slim-Fast, Slimming World, Paleo, detox plans and now Keto is the current craze. We've been told to go low fat, to go low sugar. The holiness of coconut oil was praised and then put in the realm of the darkest of poisons.

What diet is the best?
Which one really works?
If it's weight loss you're after, well, they can all help you achieve that short term. Any calorie-restricted program will. But, is it still considered effective if it only works for six months? A year? Five years? At what point do you say the diet worked?

Often when you inevitably quit the diet, our culture teaches you to blame yourself, your lack of willpower or self-control. But, if a diet works… shouldn't you be able to stick to it for life? Wouldn't it actually be the diet's fault if it causes you to 'break'? To say "I just want some freaking carbs"?

So, is there a diet that works for good? Sure is. I'm currently on it.

What's the magic formula? In my experience it has to tick the following boxes:

☑ It's accessible to your current budget, family needs, time restraints and lifestyle.

☑ It makes you feel good!

☑ It's both physically and mentally sustainable.

Let me elaborate:
It's accessible: All our lives are different. Some have families of five, some are single. Some of us have a $250 budget for groceries each week, some have $25. Some of us travel often, some work from home.

So any way of eating that you take on has to fit within your current situation. If your diet is causing you financial stress then it's not sustainable. If it's too hard to find certain foods on the road and your job requires you to travel, it's not sustainable. If you are exhausted following a busy day at work and have to spend an extra 45 minutes each night making something that you can fit into your plan, while your family sticks to the usual. That may not be sustainable either.

A way of eating that lasts has to be flexible or else, you guessed it – it won't last or won't even be doable, to begin with.

It makes you feel good. Physically AND mentally. Most diets, when you start them, do in fact make you feel great. If they don't, as I have said before, they are not sustainable. But you have to remember that health is more than how your body feels. Health is also about how you feel mentally and emotionally. If your diet causes you to feel left out, craving your favourite foods, or any kind of stress at all when it comes to eating out or visiting friends and family then it's not as healthy as you'd like to think, and eventually the cravings become too much and the cycle of 'on again off again' continues.

It's sustainable. I know, I keep hammering on about this but seriously – for any diet to work it simply has to be adherable.

The way of eating that you choose has to allow for enjoyment. If you feel deprived in any way, or miss your favourite foods or think "I wish I could eat that". Then eventually you will crave and cave. It happens almost every single time.

You may think you're not deprived. Those coconut flour buns might hold you over for now but if you genuinely love a good quality baked bread and have put it in the 'naughty' list, eventually you're going to have some and the feelings that follow that will decide the outcome.

Not only that, but any diet you choose should not only be sustainable mentally but also physically sustainable. In some cases you may be able to go for quite a long time on a nutrient deficient diet but eventually it will catch up with you. As you've learned, your body needs proteins, healthy fats, fibre, and all those delicious little micronutrients. Eventually, a lack in these vital elements that make you healthy, is going to turn that "I feel great" feeling into the opposite. You are human and there are certain things a human being needs to function optimally.

So what's the best diet on the planet? Not being on a diet! Simply eating in a way that is accessible, enjoyable and sustainable and provides a variety of nutrients considering your current budget/lifestyle. One that enables you to have a piece of cake or freshly baked bread (or whatever else you love to eat) and move on.

One that understands that health is a feeling, not a look. Healthy eating has to be flexible, enjoyable, compassionate, sustainable, simple and delicious. If it leaves you feeling deprived, even if it's six months down the road, then you're simply not going to be able to adhere to it and that's not a weakness.

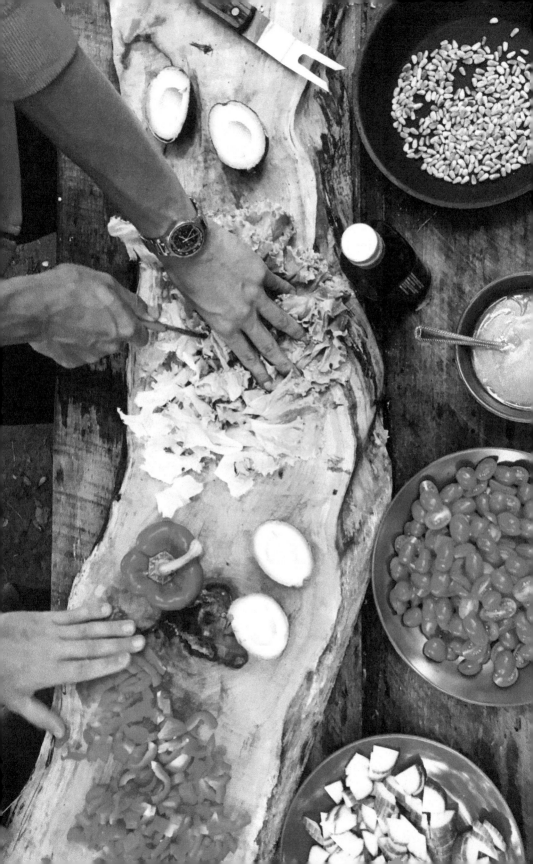

Meal Planning
Made Simple

So, you may wonder, if I'm eating intuitively and ditching the diets doesn't that mean I have to ditch the meal prep and planning too?

Absolutely not. It all boils down to intention. When done from the correct space, meal planning is a form of self-care rather than self-control. It's about making your life easier so that you can think less about food and more about getting on with your day and doing what you love.

It's about getting away from rules, calorie counting, rigidity, and making you feel like you've blown it if you go off the plan. And embracing meal planning as a way to reduce stress, budget, remembering what to put in your cart and nourishing yourself. The trick is, that you have to do it for yourself!

So, how do you meal plan? Well, to be honest, like all things, there is no one way to do a meal plan. I may do mine very differently than what works for you. And sometimes my meal plan doesn't go to plan at all. Sometimes I leave out 2-3 days on the plan (mostly on weekends) which allows flexibility if we want to go out to eat, or have to use up what we've already got in the house.

Sunday is my shopping day so meal planning for me starts on Monday. I love looking at recipes online and in books, so throughout the week, whenever I see a recipe I like on Facebook or Instagram, I save it. There's even a little button on both that allows you to do this. Otherwise, if I see it on the web there are a couple places that I will store them. Pinterest is still one of my favourites and then there is also a great program called Plan To Eat that also does up handy-dandy shopping lists.

So, by Saturday, I usually have some new recipes to try along with some favourites. If you already have some favourites, start there and then you can just keep adding to your favourites list as you go.

It doesn't have to be difficult, time-consuming or rigid. Use meal planning as a base-line, have the ingredients on hand, and it is so much easier to nourish your body.

When writing my plan, there's nothing fancy about it. Basically I keep things simple by having themed nights, but there's no hard rule with this.

It may look something like this:

Sunday is fish (I get it fresh at the market),

Monday we have beef,

Tuesday is chicken,

Wednesday is soup (salad in summer),

Thursday is vegetarian,

Friday is usually a whole roasted chicken from the supermarket and bagged salad (usually don't feel like cooking by then) or just grabbing whatever we have left.

Saturday is a "flexi-day" so either making something up with what's in the fridge or using leftovers.

I also save my favourite meals by writing them down on my computer or in a book. That way I can remember the ones my family loved and go back to them whenever I need them. Some people just stick to the same thing every week with little flexibility and if that works for you, that's fine too! I love experimenting with new recipes.

I also have to think about when I'm working late. So for example, Monday's used to be a late night for me so I would pick out something simple that my husband could make (sorry honey) or at least get started. On Friday's I'm usually just about over it so that's when I get the good old reliable ready-roasted chicken and salad meal.

Now, as far as the logistics, I just draw some columns based on the store or by grouping ingredients and scribble what I plan to eat on the other side. I go through each recipe that I have chosen and read through the ingredients, as soon as I find an ingredient that I don't have, I write it in the appropriate column.

When it comes to breakfast, I usually stick to my favourites and keep the ingredients handy. You can write you ideas down for breakfast of course but unless I'm trying something new, I don't do this. Breakfast for me is either a blueberry smoothie, oats, or toast on the weekend. As long as I've got the staples; blueberries, almond milk, eggs, oats, sourdough, peanut butter, protein powder, I can make a variety of breakfasts.

I choose one or two snack recipes, such as protein balls or bliss balls, to make also but you don't need to. You could just write down some favourite snacks onto your shopping list (nuts, fruit, muesli bars, yoghurt etc) and keep them on hand.

What about lunch? I'm going to be the first to admit that lunch can be tricky. That's why I try hard to make a little bit extra at dinner time so that both my husband and I have some leftovers for lunch. These are my go-to most days of the week and on other days I'm usually grabbing a salad at my local healthy food establishments. Otherwise scrambled eggs it another easy favourite.

This probably sounds really complicated but trust me when I say – I wouldn't do it this way if it was. The entire thing probably takes about 30 minutes or less of total planning time on a Saturday night before shopping day.

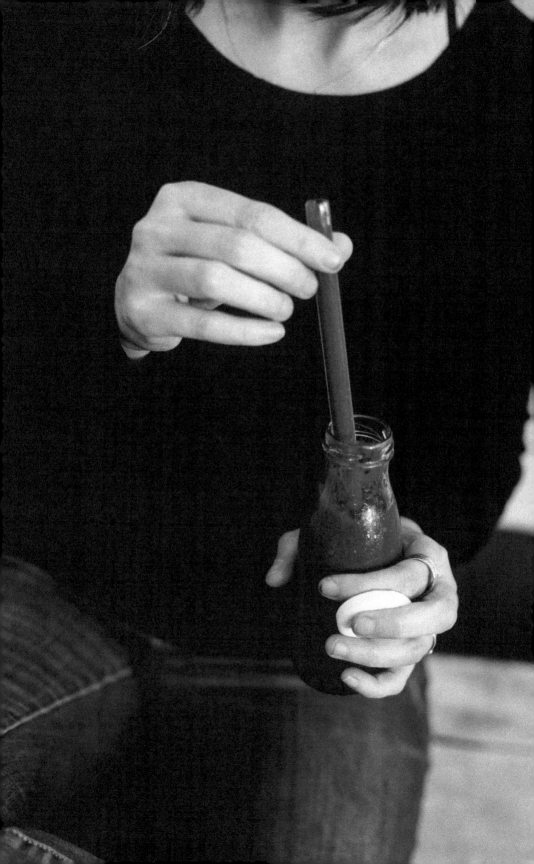

Recipes *to Inspire*

Berry Beauty**

INGREDIENTS

1 cup romaine or cos lettice
1 cup kale
1 ½ cup water or milk of choice
½ cup strawberries
½ avocado
1 tablespoon ground flax seeds
Add pea protein (vanilla) or ½ banana
to sweeten.

Sweet Sunshine**

INGREDIENTS

1 cup spinach or kale
1 peeled orange
1 ½ cups water or milk of choice
½ cup frozen berries
1 tablespoon raw cacao
½ frozen banana

Green Madness**

INGREDIENTS

1 cup water or milk of choice
1 banana, frozen
½ avocado
Handful of parsley
1 cup kale or baby spinach
1 tablespoon ground flax seeds
1 tablespoon chia seeds
1 teaspoon cinnamon
½ teaspoon vanilla (optional)
Stevia to taste
3 to 4 ice cubes

Spinach and Pumpkin Power**

INGREDIENTS

1 cup water or milk of choice
3 tablespoons pumpkin seeds
1 small frozen banana, sliced into
2-inch chunks
1 cup frozen blueberries
1 cup spinach
1 tablespoon ground flax seeds
1 tablespoon chia seeds
1 teaspoon cinnamon
Stevia to taste
3 to 4 ice cubes (optional)

**INSTRUCTIONS FOR ALL SMOOTHIES

Mix together in a blender. Add water to reach your desired smoothie thickness.
Each serving is for 2 people or 1 large meal substitute.

Fig Power**

INGREDIENTS

1 ½ cups milk of choice
3-4 fresh figs, washed, stems removed, and halved
1 frozen banana
1 cup spinach
1 teaspoon cinnamon
1 tablespoon chia seeds or flax seeds
3 to 4 ice cubes

Super Energy**

INGREDIENTS

2 cups spinach
1 ½ cups water or milk of choice
½ cup frozen mango
1 tablespoon ground flax seeds
1 teaspoon chia seeds
1 scoop protein powder or ½ banana +
¼ cup cashews

Chocolate Kale**

INGREDIENTS

1 cup milk of choice
1 frozen banana
1 cup of kale
3 tablespoons of cacao nibs
1 tablespoon of raw cacao
5 to 6 ice cubes

Chocolate Berry Bomb**

INGREDIENTS

½ cup frozen berries(fresh optional)
1 ½ cups water or milk of choice
2 cups spinach
handful of parsley
1 teaspoon raw cacao
½ teaspoon cinnamon
1 teaspoon honey or 1-2 drops liquid stevia
1 tablespoon unsweetened shredded coconut (optional topping)

Kale is King**

INGREDIENTS

2 cups kale
1 ½ cups water or milk of choice
1 cup frozen berries
1 teaspoon honey or 1-2 drops liquid stevia
1 teaspoon ground flax seeds
1 scoop of your favourite protein powder or a handful of nuts.

**INSTRUCTIONS FOR ALL SMOOTHIES

Mix together in a blender. Add water to reach your desired smoothie thickness.
Each serving is for 2 people or 1 large meal substitute.

Apple Chia Seed Pudding

Makes 2 servings

2 cups unsweetened non-dairy milk such as almond or coconut

½ teaspoon vanilla extract

2/3 cup chia seeds

2 tablespoons unsweetened coconut flakes

2 apples, cored and chopped

2 teaspoons cinnamon

For warm chia seed pudding, place your milk and vanilla extract into a saucepan, and warm over low heat for 2 to 3 minutes. The milk does not have to be boiling hot, just warm enough for your taste. Add your chia seeds to a cereal bowl. When the milk is warm, add the milk to your bowl of chia seeds. Stir continuously for about 2 minutes while the chia seeds absorb the milk. Allow the mixture to sit for 2 to 3 minutes. Top with coconut flakes, apple slices, and cinnamon.

Note: If you do NOT want warm chia seed pudding, simply add the milk to your bowl of chia seeds. Stir until the chia seeds have absorbed the milk (about 3 to 5 minutes). Then top with coconut flakes, apples, and cinnamon.

Warm Chia Breakfast Pudding

1 cup dairy-free milk of your choice (coconut, almond or hemp)

1/3 cup chia seeds

1 teaspoon vanilla extract (optional)

Assemble the night before. The night before you want the pudding for breakfast, mix the milk, chia seeds, and vanilla if using in a container with a lid. Shake well and let it sit overnight in the refrigerator. The next morning, transfer the chia pudding from the container to a pot on the stove. Warm it for 2 to 3 minutes and serve it in a bowl.

Serving suggestion: Add a sweetener of your choice. Top with dried apricots, pomegranate seeds, sliced apple or pear, etc.

Scrambled Eggs with Spinach and Peppers

Makes 2 servings

INGREDIENTS

1 tablespoon olive oil
½ cup chopped red capsicum
1 cup baby spinach
Pinch of oregano
Sea salt to taste
Black pepper to taste
2 eggs, beaten

INSTRUCTIONS

Add your oil to a hot skillet and allow it to melt. Add chopped red bell pepper and allow it to soften. After about 2 to 3 minutes, add baby spinach. The spinach should quickly wilt. Season with oregano, sea salt, and black pepper. Next, add the beaten eggs to the vegetables. Tilt the pan so the eggs spread out evenly. Use a rubber scraper or spatula to turn the eggs over so that they don't harden and burn. Scramble the eggs for 2 to 3 minutes to your desired consistency. Serve with your favourite grainy bread.

Spanish Eggs

Makes 4 servings

INGREDIENTS

8 eggs
2 cups of your favourite tomato based pasta sauce.
Goat cheese or another favourite cheese to sprinkle
Fresh parsley

INSTRUCTIONS

Preheat oven to 180°C.

Place ½ cup tomato sauce into each of 4 ramekins. Crack two organic eggs on top of the tomato sauce in each ramekin. Place in the oven and cook until the eggs begin to harden.

Remove the eggs from the oven and sprinkle with goat cheese or your favourite full fat cheese. Sprinkle with parsley. Cook until the eggs are puffy and beginning to brown on the top. Allow to cool for a few minutes then serve.

Lemon Pancakes

Makes 1-2 servings

INGREDIENTS

½ cup almond flour/meal (or simply grind up your nuts of choice)
2 eggs (organic and/or free range)
½ banana
1 teaspoon cinnamon
½ teaspoon vanilla extract
1 tablespoon linseed/ground flaxseed
Zest from 1 lemon.
(a little almond milk if needed)

Olive oil or butter for cooking

INSTRUCTIONS

Whizz all the ingredients in a blender and then pour into your hot oil or butter-greased pan. Cook until you start to see the bubbles burst on the top and then cook on the other side until done.

Grain-Free Porridge

INGREDIENTS

¼ cup raw pumpkin seeds
2 tablespoons flax seeds
1 tablespoon chia seeds
2 tablespoons unsweetened shredded coconut
1 teaspoon cinnamon
½ teaspoon ginger
½ teaspoon vanilla extract
½ cup warm dairy-free milk of your choice

INSTRUCTIONS

Grind the cereal. In a coffee grinder or blender, add the pumpkin seeds, flax seeds, chia seeds, and shredded coconut. Grind or blend until fine. Place in a serving bowl. Add warm dairy-free milk along with cinnamon, ginger, and vanilla.

Serving Suggestions. Add spices like cinnamon, allspice, ginger, or garam masala to your cereal. Or you may add a teaspoon of the sweetener of your choice. Top your cereal with sliced bananas, apples, shredded coconut, etc.

Kale with Apple Salad

4 cups of kale, thinly sliced
1 cup parsley, chopped
1 large lemon, juiced
1 avocado, chopped
4 tablespoons extra virgin olive oil
¼ teaspoon sea salt
¼ teaspoon black pepper
1 large apple, chopped
¼ cup carrots, shredded

Add kale, parsley, lemon juice, avocado, oil, sea salt, and black pepper to a large bowl. Massage the kale and other ingredients with clean hands. The kale should turn a bright green and become softer. Taste and adjust seasoning as needed.

Add remaining ingredients. Toss and top with pumpkin seeds and dried cranberries if desired.

Mean Green Wrap with Sunflower Seeds

Makes 2 servings

Sunflower Seed Pate
1 cup sunflower seeds, soaked overnight
1 large tomato
¼ bunch coriander
2 to 3 sundried tomatoes
3 tablespoons extra virgin olive oil
2 tablespoons tahini
2 lemons, juiced
Sea salt

Black pepper

Pate Topping Options
1 cup cultured vegetables, sprouts, shredded carrots, shredded leftover chicken, canned salmon or smoked salmon

Drain the water from the sunflower seeds and place the seeds in a food processor or blender. Add the remaining ingredients and blend until smooth. Add 1 to 2 tablespoons of water to get desired consistency, if needed.Season to taste.

To assemble your wrap, add 2 to 3 tablespoons of pate to your chosen wrap. Add desired toppings. Roll it up and enjoy.

**You can also use romaine lettuce, a collard leaf, a nori sheet, or your favourite wheat based or gluten free wrap as a wrap for this recipe.

Chopped Beauty Salad with Tahini Dressing

Makes 2 servings

INGREDIENTS

2 cups spinach

2 cups thinly sliced purple cabbage

½ bunch flat leaf parsley, chopped

½ cup shredded carrots

1 large cucumber, chopped
into pieces

5 to 6 mint leaves, minced

Tahini Dressing

½ cup tahini

2 lemons, juiced

1 Tbsp honey t

3/4 to 1 cup of water

1 large garlic clove, minced

Sea salt

Black pepper

INSTRUCTIONS

Add your dressing ingredients to a jar with a lid. Shake vigorously and allow the flavors to marinate while you prepare the salad. Add your salad ingredients to a large serving bowl. Toss with the Tahini Dressing. Season to taste. Top with your favourite protein – grilled chicken, canned fish, chicpeas or hard boiled eggs.

Roasted Winter Vegetables

INGREDIENTS

2 large parsnips, peeled and chopped

2 small beetroot, peeled and
chopped

250g pumpkin chopped

2 tablespoons extra virgin olive oil

1 teaspoon garlic powder

¼ bunch parsley, minced

Sea salt

Black pepper

INSTRUCTIONS

Preheat the oven. Preheat the oven to 180°C. Roast your vegetables. Place your parsnips, beets, and pumpkin into a roasting pan. Add extra virgin olive oil, garlic powder, sea salt, and black pepper. Roast for 40 to 45 minutes. When the vegetables are tender, remove from the oven and let it cool for 5 minutes. Top with minced parsley to serve. Enjoy!

Roasted Summer Vegetables

Makes 3 to 4 servings

INGREDIENTS

2 large red onions, roughly chopped into bite sized pieces
1 cup chopped zucchini
1 cup chopped pumpkin
1 cup chopped carrot
1 cup chopped red capsicum
2 cups chopped eggplant
1 tablespoon dried rosemary
1 tablespoon thyme
2 tablespoons olive oil
Sea salt to taste

INSTRUCTIONS

Preheat your oven to 180°C. Add your chopped vegetables, rosemary, thyme, and oil to a large mixing bowl. Toss until well coated. Spread your vegetables onto a roasting pan into a single layer. Roast the vegetables for 30 to 35 minutes. The vegetables should be browned and tender. Add sea salt and mix thoroughly.

Add your favourite protein on the side.

Sweet and Spicy Collard Slaw

INGREDIENTS

1 bunch collard greens, thinly sliced
½ small red cabbage, thinly sliced
1 large carrot, shredded
½ teaspoon red pepper flakes (optional)

Dressing

2 oranges, juiced
¼ cup raw apple cider vinegar (omit if you have acid reflux)
½ cup extra virgin olive oil
2 teaspoons powdered cumin
1 date, pitted
1 small garlic clove
Sea salt
Black pepper

INSTRUCTIONS

Prepare the dressing first to allow the flavors to intermingle. Add the orange juice, raw apple cider vinegar, oil, cumin, the pitted date, garlic clove, sea salt, and black pepper to a blender. Blend until smooth. Taste and adjust seasonings to your preference. Allow the dressing to sit for at least 15 minutes.

Toss the salad. Add your thinly sliced collards, red cabbage, and carrot to a large salad bowl. Add enough dressing to coat the salad, but not drown it. Add red pepper flakes if desired. Mix thoroughly. Enjoy!

Romaine with Mango Basil Dressing

Makes 2 servings

INGREDIENTS

2 heads romaine or cos lettuce, chopped
1 cup cherry tomatoes
½ cup coriander, chopped
1 cup chopped red pepper
¼ cup chopped purple cabbage
½ cup chopped cucumbers
2 tablespoons pumpkin seeds

Mango-Basil Dressing

1 cup fresh mango, chopped
1 lime, juiced
5 to 6 basil leaves
½ cup extra virgin olive oil
Pinch of sea salt
Pinch of black pepper

INSTRUCTIONS

Assemble your salad. Add your dressing ingredients to a blender and blend until smooth. Add to your salad. Top with your favourite protein. Cashew nuts are lovely on this.

Herb Salad

INGREDIENTS

1 head broccoli, chopped into bite-sized pieces
½ head cauliflower, chopped into bite-sized pieces
1 large carrot, shredded
1 pear, chopped
¼ cup minced red onion
½ bunch coriander, minced
½ bunch dill, minced
½ bunch mint leaves, minced

Dressing

2 lemons, juiced
¼ cup raw apple cider vinegar
¼ cup extra virgin olive oil
Sea salt
Black pepper

INSTRUCTIONS

Prepare the dressing first to allow the flavors to intermingle. Add the lemon juice, raw apple cider vinegar and oil, to a container with a lid. Shake vigorously until well blended.Season with salt and pepper and adjust to your preference. Allow to sit for at least 15 minutes.

Chop the broccoli and cauliflower into small bite sized pieces for easier digestion. Add to a large salad bowl along with shredded carrot, chopped pear, red onion, cilantro, dill, and mint. Add enough dressing to coat the salad, but not drown it. Mix thoroughly. If desired add any of these suggested toppings: diced avocado, dried cranberry, and sprouts. Enjoy!

Mediterranean Salad

2 cups mesclun lettuce

1 cup flat leaf parsley, chopped

1 carrot, shredded

1 large apple, chopped

¼ cup shredded beetroot

10 fresh mint leaves, roughly torn to small pieces

1 avocado, chopped

Kalamata olives, chopped (optional)

Dressing

2 large garlic cloves, minced

1 large lemon, juiced

¼ cup red wine vinegar

¼ cup extra virgin olive oil

½ teaspoon dijon mustard

1 teaspoon dried oregano

Sea salt

Black pepper

Prepare the dressing first to allow the flavors to intermingle. Add all the ingredients to a jar with a lid. Shake vigorously. Taste and adjust seasonings to your preference. Allow the dressing to sit for at least 15 minutes.

Toss the salad. Add your mesclun lettuce, parsley, apple, beetroot, and mint leaves to a large salad bowl. Add enough dressing to coat the salad, but not drown it. Mix thoroughly. Top with chopped avocado and kalamata olives (optional). Enjoy!

Sweet and Sour Kale with Apricot

1 bunch kale (any variety), chopped
1 medium onion, thinly sliced
6 dried apricots, soaked and chopped
2 tablespoons apple cider vinegar
1 tablespoon extra virgin olive oil
½ teaspoon sea salt
½ teaspoon black pepper

Put apricots into a bowl with enough warm water to cover. Allow to soak for 30 minutes to 1 hour. When soft, chop into small pieces. Wash and chop kale into bite-sized pieces. Peel and slice onions into thin slices. Set aside. Set a large sauté pan on medium high heat and add oil. When hot, add the sliced onions. Sauté until soft. Add the kale and chopped apricots. Sauté until the kale is wilted and tender. Add the apple cider vinegar, sea salt and pepper. Coat the vegetables thoroughly. Turn off heat and allow the dish to marinate for 5 minutes before serving. Enjoy!

Indian Curry Cauliflower with Peas and Carrots

1 large head cauliflower
¼ cup frozen peas
¼ cup frozen carrots
2 tablespoons extra virgin olive oil
1 tablespoon curry powder
1 teaspoon mustard seeds
1 teaspoon cumin seeds
¼ teaspoon sea salt
¼ teaspoon black pepper
¼ teaspoon red pepper flakes (optional)

Preheat the oven to 200°C.
Roast the cauliflower. Wash and chop the cauliflower into bite-sized florets. Place onto a roasting pan with peas, carrots, extra virgin olive oil, curry powder, mustard seeds, cumin seeds, sea salt, black pepper, and red pepper flakes (optional). Place into a hot oven for 30 to 35 minutes. When the cauliflower is browned and tender, remove from the oven and allow to sit for 5 minutes. Place into a serving bowl. Enjoy!

Miso Soup

INGREDIENTS

5 cups water

1 strip kombu, hijiki or other sea vegetable (available at natural food stores and Bin Inns)

1 cup silverbeet, kale, or other greens, chopped

½ cup sliced carrots

5 teaspoons miso of your choice

INSTRUCTIONS

Rinse the sea vegetables in cold water for 10 minutes (if using arame, do not soak). Wipe with a towel to remove excess sodium. Fill a pot with water. Cut the sea vegetable into small strips and add to the pot. Bring the water to a boil. Add the carrots, cover and turn the heat to medium-low. Simmer for about 10 minutes. Remove a few tablespoons of broth from the pot to mix with the miso in a separate container to form a puree. Place the miso puree in the soup pot and simmer for 2 to 3 minutes (miso should not be boiled because it will kill the beneficial bacteria!). Add the greens and simmer for 2 more minutes.

Carrot Orange Spice Soup

INGREDIENTS

1 tablespoon extra virgin olive oil

1 teaspoon cumin seeds

1 small onion, chopped

1 red capsicum chopped

500g of carrots, peeled and chopped

3 cups broth (chicken or vegetable) or water

2 to 3 large oranges, juiced

INSTRUCTIONS

Create your soup base - in a large pot, add extra virgin olive oil over a medium heat. Add cumin seeds and sauté until fragrant (about 1 minute). Add chopped onion and red pepper. Sauté until soft (about 2 to 3 minutes). Add your carrots and broth (or water). Allow the soup to come to a boil. Then lower the heat to a simmer for about 10 to 15 minutes. When the carrots are tender, turn off the heat and add your orange juice. Stir until well incorporated.

Use an immersion blender to thicken the soup, or place the soup in a blender in batches and blend to your desired consistency. Add organic coconut milk if you would like your soup to be a bit more creamy.

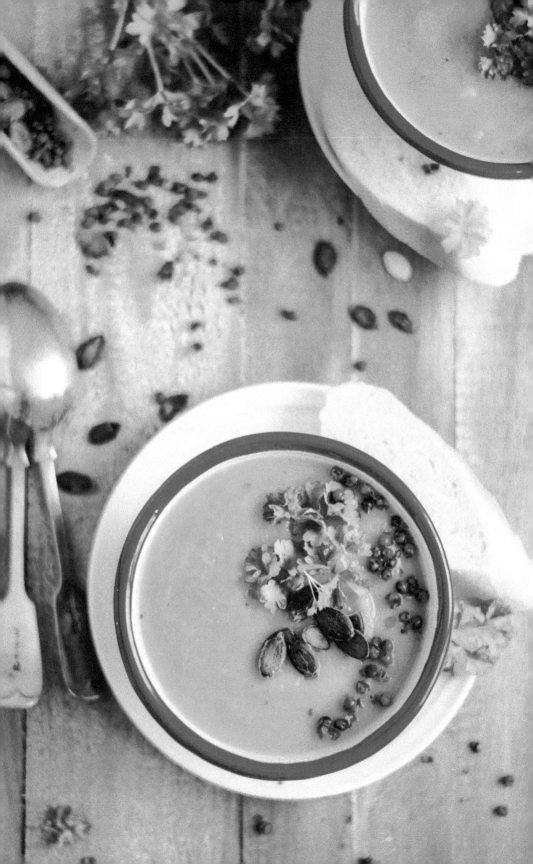

Parsnip Cream Soup

INGREDIENTS

1 tablespoon extra virgin olive oil
2 large celery ribs, chopped
1 small onion, chopped
4 large parsnips, peeled and chopped
2 teaspoons poultry or vegetable seasoning
2 cups broth (chicken or vegetable) or water
½ teaspoon sea salt
½ teaspoon black pepper
½ cup dairy-free milk of your choice (coconut, almond or hemp)

INSTRUCTIONS

In a large pot, add extra virgin olive oil on medium heat. When the pan is hot, add the celery and onion. Sauté for about 2 to 3 minutes. Add parsnips, poultry or vegetable seasoning, and broth (or water) along with sea salt and black pepper. Allow the mixture to come to a boil. Then lower the heat and simmer for 30 to 45 minutes. When the parsnips are tender, remove from heat.

Use an immersion blender or blend in batches using a standup blender to make smooth. When the soup is blended, pour it back to the pot and add the dairy-free milk. Reheat, taste and adjust seasonings. Enjoy!

Chicken Bone Broth

INGREDIENTS

1.5-3kg of soup bones*
Water (enough to cover the bones)
1 tablespoon raw apple cider vinegar
* Note: ask at your local butcher shop. Soup bones are usually very cheap, if not free!

INSTRUCTIONS

In the stock pot, add your soup bones with enough water to cover. Add apple cider vinegar. Bring to a boil, and then reduce to a simmer for 24+ hours.

Storing Stock – After about 24 hours, strain the stock into mason jars. Set them in the fridge to cool. Skim off the fat that rises to the top, and close tightly with a lid, or put in ice cube trays for quick use. Keeps in the fridge for a few days, or for four to six months in the freezer.

Chicken Soup – If you would like to make a chicken soup, add a quart of your stock to a pot with your favorite vegetables. You can use tomatoes, celery, carrots, leeks, potatoes, sweet potatoes, yams, turnips, etc. Bring to a boil, and then simmer until the vegetables are soft. Once the harder vegetables are soft, you can add chopped leafy greens like spinach, Swiss chard, or kale, if desired. Add sea salt and pepper to taste. Top with fresh herbs like parsley, basil, dill, oregano or rosemary.

Fish Fingers and Chips

Makes 3 to 4 servings

INGREDIENTS

500g of your favourite white fish.

1 cup almond meal

½ teaspoon sea salt

½ teaspoon dried parsley,
or 1 teaspoon fresh parsley

½ cup tapioca flour

2 organic free range eggs

INSTRUCTIONS

Prepare three bowls. In one bowl combine the almond meal, parsley and sea salt. In another bowl scramble the eggs. In the third bowl add the tapioca flour.

Cut your fish into strips and dip each strip one at a time into each bowl beginning with the tapioca, then the egg and finally- the almond meal mixture.

Fry the crumbed fish in a pan heated to medium heat until it is browned on all sides and cooked through.

Easy Peasy Fish Cakes

INGREDIENTS

3 cans worth of salmon, tuna or your own smoked fish.

3 organic free range eggs

¼ almond flour or macadamia meal

4 chopped spring onions

3 tablespoons of fresh squeezed lemon juice

1 tablespoon dried dill, coriander, parsley or your favourite fresh herb.

½ teaspoon ground ginger

Salt

Pepper

Olive oil to fry

INSTRUCTIONS

Add the canned or smoked fish to a large mixing bowl. Add the rest of the ingredients except for the oil.

In a large frying pan, heat the coconut oil over medium-high heat.

Meanwhile, form the mixture into small patties and place one at a time into the hot oil. Cook until browned on each side and serve with fresh guacamole and a vegetables side of choice.

Raw Corn Salad with Sautéed Salmon

Makes 4 to 5 servings

Corn Salad

6 ears of corn
1 cup chopped capsicum
1 jalapeño, diced (optional)
1 green onion, minced
½ bunch coriander, minced
1 teaspoon oregano
2 tablespoons extra virgin olive oil
Sea salt to taste

Sautéed Salmon

1-15 ounce can of salmon
1 tablespoon cumin powder
1 teaspoon paprika
½ teaspoon cayenne (optional)
1 teaspoon sea salt
1 to 2 teaspoons of olive oil
1 onion, minced
½ cup red pepper
3 cloves of garlic, minced

Corn Salad

Pull away the green from each ear of corn. Make sure to remove the silks as well. Next, get a shallow bowl and place one ear of corn inside the bowl while holding the opposite end. Using a very sharp chef's knife, gently glide the knife down the ear of corn from the top to the end. Repeat until you can get as many kernels off the ear as possible.

Add the remaining ingredients to the corn kernels and mix thoroughly.

Salmon

Open the can of salmon and dump out the water. Place the salmon in a mixing bowl and remove the large bone in the center of the fish. Use a fork to break up the fish into small pieces (as you may do with tuna fish salad). Add the cumin powder, paprika, cayenne (optional), and sea salt. Mix well.

Take a large sauté pan and add the oil. When the pan is hot, add the onion and red pepper. Sauté until soft. Next, add the minced garlic and sauté until fragrant, but not burned (about 2 minutes). Finally, add the salmon and sauté until warmed through (about 3 to 5 minutes).

Macadamia Chicken

INGREDIENTS

INGREDIENTS

4 chicken thighs

2 tablespoon olive oil or macadamia oil

½ cup macadamia nuts ground in the food processor until crumb sized

1/4 cup mayonnaise

Salt and pepper to taste

INSTRUCTIONS

Preheat oven to 180°C.

Add oil to the bottom of a rectangular baking dish. Rinse the chicken then pat dry and place in the baking dish. Spread each piece of chicken evenly with the mayonnaise then sprinkle the chicken with macadamia nut crumb and some sea salt.

Bake until the juices run clear and the macadamias have browned.

Amazingly Simple Chicken Drumsticks

INGREDIENTS

6 organic free range chicken drumsticks (leave the skins!)

1 teaspoon sweet paprika

1 teaspoongarlic powder

Salt and pepper to taste

2 tablespoon macadamia oil or olive oil

INSTRUCTIONS

Preheat oven to 180°C.

Place the oil in a rectangular baking pan, add the chicken drumsticks and toss in the oil. Sprinkle with the spices and salt and bake in the oven, turning once, until the juices run clear and the skin is crispy.

Enjoy with greens and your favourite winter veggies.

Food Diary

Remember to tune in and ask your body whether it is actually physically hungry, then follow up with asking your body what it needs. Is it food? Is it comfort? Or is it entertainment? If it's food, load up on vegetables or fruit first, add some protein and then healthy fats. Do this as often as possible and then relax and enjoy the times in between where you might want something to sooth your soul rather than your physical body.

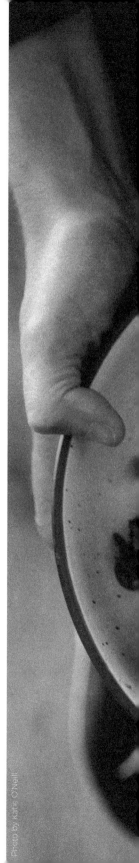

Photo by Katie O'Neill

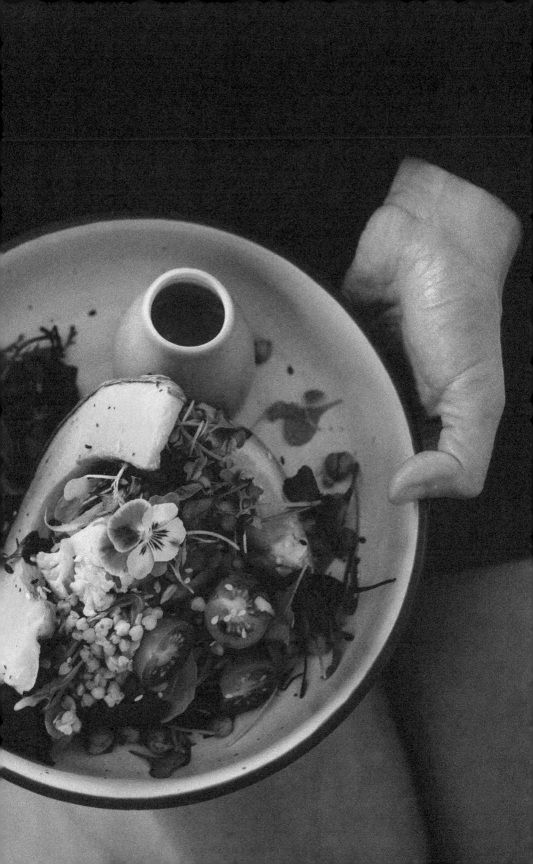

Day 1

VEGGIES AND FRUIT:

PROTEIN SOURCES:

HEALTHY FATS:

FIBRE SOURCES:

CARB SOURCES:

FERMENTED FOODS:

ONE ACT OF SELF CARE:

DRINKS:

○○○○○○○○○○
○○○○○○○○○○

TODAY I AM GRATEFUL FOR:

Day 2

VEGGIES AND FRUIT:

PROTEIN SOURCES:

HEALTHY FATS:

FIBRE SOURCES:

CARB SOURCES:

FERMENTED FOODS:

ONE ACT OF SELF CARE:

DRINKS:

○○○○○○○○○○
○○○○○○○○○○

TODAY I AM GRATEFUL FOR:

Day 3

VEGGIES AND FRUIT:

PROTEIN SOURCES:

HEALTHY FATS:

FIBRE SOURCES:

CARB SOURCES:

FERMENTED FOODS:

ONE ACT OF SELF CARE:

DRINKS:

○○○○○○○○○
○○○○○○○○○

TODAY I AM GRATEFUL FOR:

Day 4

VEGGIES AND FRUIT:

PROTEIN SOURCES:

HEALTHY FATS:

FIBRE SOURCES:

CARB SOURCES:

FERMENTED FOODS:

ONE ACT OF SELF CARE:

DRINKS:

○○○○○○○○○○
○○○○○○○○○○

TODAY I AM GRATEFUL FOR:

Day 5

VEGGIES AND FRUIT:

PROTEIN SOURCES:

HEALTHY FATS:

FIBRE SOURCES:

CARB SOURCES:

FERMENTED FOODS:

ONE ACT OF SELF CARE:

DRINKS:

○○○○○○○○○○
○○○○○○○○○○

TODAY I AM GRATEFUL FOR:

Day 6

VEGGIES AND FRUIT:

PROTEIN SOURCES:

HEALTHY FATS:

FIBRE SOURCES:

CARB SOURCES:

FERMENTED FOODS:

ONE ACT OF SELF CARE:

DRINKS:

○○○○○○○○○○
○○○○○○○○○○

TODAY I AM GRATEFUL FOR:

Day 7

VEGGIES AND FRUIT:

PROTEIN SOURCES:

HEALTHY FATS:

FIBRE SOURCES:

CARB SOURCES:

FERMENTED FOODS:

ONE ACT OF SELF CARE:

DRINKS:

◯◯◯◯◯◯◯◯◯
◯◯◯◯◯◯◯◯◯

TODAY I AM GRATEFUL FOR:

Day 8

VEGGIES AND FRUIT:

PROTEIN SOURCES:

HEALTHY FATS:

FIBRE SOURCES:

CARB SOURCES:

FERMENTED FOODS:

ONE ACT OF SELF CARE:

DRINKS:

○○○○○○○○○
○○○○○○○○○

TODAY I AM GRATEFUL FOR:

Day 9

VEGGIES AND FRUIT:

PROTEIN SOURCES:

HEALTHY FATS:

FIBRE SOURCES:

CARB SOURCES:

FERMENTED FOODS:

ONE ACT OF SELF CARE:

DRINKS:

○○○○○○○○○
○○○○○○○○○

TODAY I AM GRATEFUL FOR:

WELCOME
HEALTH. LOVE
AND
HAPPINESS INTO
YOUR LIFE.
———

Day 10

VEGGIES AND FRUIT:

PROTEIN SOURCES:

HEALTHY FATS:

FIBRE SOURCES:

CARB SOURCES:

FERMENTED FOODS:

ONE ACT OF SELF CARE:

DRINKS:

○○○○○○○○○○
○○○○○○○○○○

TODAY I AM GRATEFUL FOR:

Day 11

VEGGIES AND FRUIT:

PROTEIN SOURCES:

HEALTHY FATS:

FIBRE SOURCES:

CARB SOURCES:

FERMENTED FOODS:

ONE ACT OF SELF CARE:

DRINKS:

○○○○○○○○○○
○○○○○○○○○○

TODAY I AM GRATEFUL FOR:

Day 12

VEGGIES AND FRUIT:

PROTEIN SOURCES:

HEALTHY FATS:

FIBRE SOURCES:

CARB SOURCES:

FERMENTED FOODS:

ONE ACT OF SELF CARE:

DRINKS:

◯◯◯◯◯◯◯◯◯◯
◯◯◯◯◯◯◯◯◯◯

TODAY I AM GRATEFUL FOR:

Day 13

VEGGIES AND FRUIT:

PROTEIN SOURCES:

HEALTHY FATS:

FIBRE SOURCES:

CARB SOURCES:

FERMENTED FOODS:

ONE ACT OF SELF CARE:

DRINKS:

○○○○○○○○○○
○○○○○○○○○○

TODAY I AM GRATEFUL FOR:

Day 14

VEGGIES AND FRUIT:

PROTEIN SOURCES:

HEALTHY FATS:

FIBRE SOURCES:

CARB SOURCES:

FERMENTED FOODS:

ONE ACT OF SELF CARE:

DRINKS:

○○○○○○○○○
○○○○○○○○○

TODAY I AM GRATEFUL FOR:

Day 15

VEGGIES AND FRUIT:

PROTEIN SOURCES:

HEALTHY FATS:

FIBRE SOURCES:

CARB SOURCES:

FERMENTED FOODS:

ONE ACT OF SELF CARE:

DRINKS:

OOOOOOOOOO
OOOOOOOOOO

TODAY I AM GRATEFUL FOR:

Day 16

VEGGIES AND FRUIT:

PROTEIN SOURCES:

HEALTHY FATS:

FIBRE SOURCES:

CARB SOURCES:

FERMENTED FOODS:

ONE ACT OF SELF CARE:

DRINKS:

○○○○○○○○○○
○○○○○○○○○○

TODAY I AM GRATEFUL FOR:

Day 17

VEGGIES AND FRUIT:

PROTEIN SOURCES:

HEALTHY FATS:

FIBRE SOURCES:

CARB SOURCES:

FERMENTED FOODS:

ONE ACT OF SELF CARE:

DRINKS:

○○○○○○○○○○
○○○○○○○○○○

TODAY I AM GRATEFUL FOR:

Day 18

VEGGIES AND FRUIT:

PROTEIN SOURCES:

HEALTHY FATS:

FIBRE SOURCES:

CARB SOURCES:

FERMENTED FOODS:

ONE ACT OF SELF CARE:

DRINKS:

○○○○○○○○○○
○○○○○○○○○○

TODAY I AM GRATEFUL FOR:

Day 19

VEGGIES AND FRUIT:

PROTEIN SOURCES:

HEALTHY FATS:

FIBRE SOURCES:

CARB SOURCES:

FERMENTED FOODS:

ONE ACT OF SELF CARE:

DRINKS:

OOOOOOOOOO
OOOOOOOOOO

TODAY I AM GRATEFUL FOR:

Day 20

VEGGIES AND FRUIT:

PROTEIN SOURCES:

HEALTHY FATS:

FIBRE SOURCES:

CARB SOURCES:

FERMENTED FOODS:

ONE ACT OF SELF CARE:

DRINKS:

○○○○○○○○○○
○○○○○○○○○○

TODAY I AM GRATEFUL FOR:

Day 21

VEGGIES AND FRUIT:

PROTEIN SOURCES:

HEALTHY FATS:

FIBRE SOURCES:

CARB SOURCES:

FERMENTED FOODS:

ONE ACT OF SELF CARE:

DRINKS:

○○○○○○○○○○
○○○○○○○○○○

TODAY I AM GRATEFUL FOR:

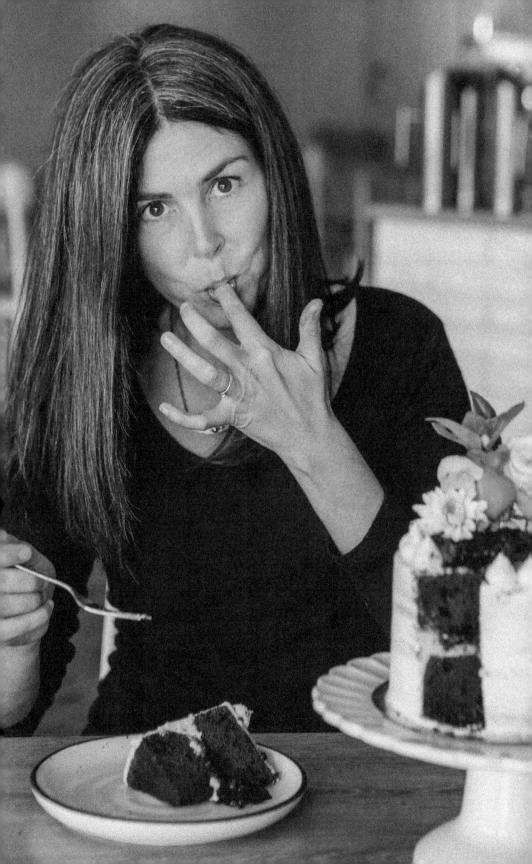

About the Author
Michelle Yandle

Nutrition Coach. Healthy Food Ambassador.
Teacher. Author. Cat Lover. Recovered Yo-Yo Dieter.

A certified Health and Nutrition Coach, Michelle Yandle is also an international speaker with IISB, successful entrepreneur, Empowered Eating™ coach and two-time author with a focus on traditional diets for health, and nutrition coaching for Empowered Eating™.

Originally from Canada, Michelle received her bachelor degree at Dalhousie University, Halifax while later achieving a graduate degree in education at the University of Maine at Fort Kent. She then furthered her education with a graduate certificate through the school of Holistic Performance Nutrition and certificates in health and nutrition coaching from the Institute for Integrative Nutrition and Cadence Health in New Zealand.

Michelle's health advice has featured in such magazines as *Nadia Magazine* and *Healthy Food Guide*. She has been a guest blogger at AwesoME Inc® – where this series on Gentle Nutrition was first published, as well as Ecostore, Elephant Journal, NZ Woman and more. She has also been a guest on The Hitz Radio and The AM Show, a regular feature in local and national newspapers and is an author and National Ambassador for Nuzest New Zealand.

For more information:
www.MichelleYandle.com
 michelleyandlenutrition

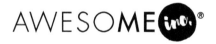

A Guide to Gentle Nutrition is published by AwesoME Inc®
– the place to go to source the tools, backed by science, to help
improve your happiness and well-being.

For more information about AwesoME Inc®, our awesome
programmes and products, including books, gratitude journals,
resilience training, vision board templates, prints and postcards go to:

WWW.AWESOMEENDSIN.ME

 AwesomeEndsInMe   awesomeinc_nz

CPSIA information can be obtained
at www.ICGtesting.com
Printed in the USA
LVHW072102090820
662765LV00042B/1194